Nutshell Guide for MRCOG Part 2

Managing Problems of Early Pregnancy Module

Authors: Peter Hanna, Mohammed Gaber, Mina Younan

KEYPOINTS REVISION, 200 SBA
& 70 EMQ QUESTIONS

Contents

Introduction to the Authors: 3

Preface 5

Early Pregnancy Assessment Services and Pregnancy of Unknown Location 11

    Single Best Answer (SBA) Questions 14

    Extended Match Questions (EMQ) 22

Ectopic Pregnancy: A Comprehensive Overview 33

    Cervical Ectopic Pregnancy 37

    Caesarean Section Scar Ectopic Pregnancy (CSP) Summary 39

    Single Best Answer (SBA) Questions 42

    Extended Match Questions (EMQ) 61

Early Pregnancy Ultrasound 69

    Single Best Answer (SBA) Questions 73

    Extended Match Questions (EMQ) 98

Anti-D Prophylaxis 116

    Single Best Answer (SBA) Questions 118

    Extended Match Questions (EMQ) 125

Recurrent Miscarriage 134

    Single Best Answer Questions: 137

    Extended Match Questions (EMQ) 144

.Nausea and Vomiting in Pregnancy NVP, and Hyperemesis Gravidarum (HG) 152

    Single Best Answer Questions: 156

    Extended Match Questions (EMQ) 168

Answers 178

Single Best Answer (SBA): Answers 179

Extended Match Questions (EMQ) Answers 213

Introduction to the Authors:

Dr. Peter Hanna and **Dr. Mohammed Gaber** are members of the Royal College of Obstetricians and Gynaecologists (RCOG) who have dedicated their careers to advancing medical knowledge and supporting their peers.

Dr. Peter Hanna is a committed Specialty Registrar with a postgraduate degree in Medical Education. His expertise lies in applying the latest clinical evidence, RCOG, and NICE guidelines to develop high-quality educational materials. His passion for education is reflected in his significant contributions to this book, where he has meticulously gathered evidence, created comprehensive study notes, and crafted challenging MRCOG exam questions.

Dr. Mohammed Gaber, with his MRCOG, MSc, and EBCOG qualifications, brings his experience as an ST3 in Obstetrics and Gynaecology at Tameside and Glossop Integrated Care NHS Foundation Trust. His deep understanding of clinical practice, coupled with his commitment to teaching, has been instrumental in shaping this resource.

Together, Dr. Hanna and Dr. Gaber have pooled their extensive knowledge and experience to create a practical and comprehensive guide designed to help candidates excel in the MRCOG Part 2 exam preparation.

Dr Mina Younan, MBBCh. MRCS., is a Speciality Doctor in General Surgery who helped greatly to provide ideas and revise the questions and the delivery of the book. Their shared commitment to education and excellence in obstetrics and gynaecology is evident in the quality and depth of the content, making this book an invaluable tool for aspiring specialists.

Preface

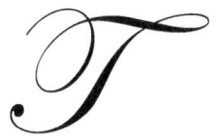his book is the culmination of dedication, passion, and the invaluable support of those closest to me.

 I would like to express my deepest gratitude to my wife, Madonna, for her unwavering encouragement, and to my two daughters, Adora and Alora, whose love and joy inspire me every day. I am also deeply thankful to Dr. Dr Gaber and Dr Younan, whose expertise and insightful contributions were instrumental in shaping this work. This book would not have been possible without your collective support and belief in its purpose.

Peter Hanna, August 2024

Introduction

Embarking on the journey to obtain your MRCOG qualification is a significant milestone in your career as an obstetrician and gynaecologist. The Part 2 MRCOG exam, with its rigorous testing of your clinical knowledge, judgement, and decision-making abilities, represents a critical step in this journey. This book has been meticulously crafted to support you in this endeavour, offering a comprehensive and focused resource designed specifically for your exam preparation.

The book you hold in your hands is the result of a collaborative effort between three dedicated professionals, Dr. Peter Hanna, Dr Mohammed Gaber and Dr Mina Younan, who bring their extensive experience in exam preparation and deep commitment to the advancement of medical education to this project.

This book contains 200 Single Best Answer (SBA) questions and 70 stem Extended Matching Questions (EMQs), each carefully designed to cover the spectrum of early pregnancy care problems. The questions are intended to test your knowledge, clinical reasoning, and application of guidelines in scenarios that are commonly encountered in the exam. In addition to these questions, the book provides concise summaries of key topics. These summaries are crafted to help you quickly recall important information and reinforce your understanding before tackling the questions.

Preparing for the Part 2 MRCOG exam requires not just knowledge, but also strategy. Here are some study tips to help you maximise your preparation:

1. **Create a Study Plan:** Structure your study time with a clear schedule. Allocate sufficient time to each topic area, ensuring you cover all aspects of the syllabus.

2. **Active Learning:** Engage with the material actively. Use the questions in this book to test your knowledge regularly. Don't just passively read the summaries—apply what you've learned by answering the questions.

3. **Review and Reflect:** After answering the questions, take the time to review the explanations and identify

areas where you need further study. Reflect on your mistakes as opportunities to improve.

4. **Simulate Exam Conditions:** Practice answering questions under timed conditions. This will help you manage your time effectively during the actual exam and reduce anxiety.

5. **Stay Updated:** The field of obstetrics and gynaecology is constantly evolving. Stay informed about the latest guidelines and evidence, as these can influence the correct answers in your exam.

We wish you the best of luck in your preparation. Remember, the MRCOG exam is not just a test of knowledge, but a demonstration of your ability to apply that knowledge in clinical practice. With determination, consistent effort, and the resources provided in this book, you are well on your way to success.

How to Use This Book

This book is designed to be a practical and comprehensive tool for your MRCOG Part 2 exam preparation. To make the most of it, start by familiarising yourself with the summaries provided for each key topic. These summaries are concise yet comprehensive, offering you a solid foundation of knowledge that you can build upon as you study.

Next, use the SBA and EMQ questions to test your understanding and application of the material. Each question has been crafted to reflect the style and difficulty of the actual MRCOG exam. After answering, review the explanations carefully, even for questions you answered correctly. This will help you reinforce your knowledge and correct any misconceptions.

It is recommended that you integrate these questions into your daily study routine, rather than saving them all for a single session. This approach allows for spaced repetition, which is proven to enhance memory retention. Additionally, as you work through the questions, take note of any areas where you consistently struggle, and revisit those topics in the summaries.

By using this book consistently and strategically, you can build the confidence and competence needed to excel in the Part 2 MRCOG exam.

Good luck, and may your efforts lead to success.

Peter Hanna
August 2024

Early Pregnancy Assessment Services and Pregnancy of Unknown Location

Early Pregnancy Assessment Services

1. **Service Availability**:
   - Early pregnancy assessment services should be accessible **7 days a week**.
2. **Healthcare Professional Competency**:
   - Services should be provided by professionals trained to **diagnose and care for women experiencing pain and/or bleeding in early pregnancy**.
   - They should be capable of performing **ultrasound scans** and **assessing serum human chorionic gonadotrophin (hCG) levels**.
   - Staff should also be trained in **sensitive communication** and **breaking bad news**.
3. **Referral Protocol**:
   - **Self-referral** is allowed for women with a history of **recurrent miscarriage**, **previous ectopic pregnancy**, or **molar pregnancy**.
   - Other women with pain and/or bleeding should first be assessed by a **healthcare**

- **professional** (GP, A&E doctor, midwife, nurse) before being referred.
  - If the early pregnancy assessment service is unavailable and clinical symptoms require urgent attention, women should be referred to the **nearest facility** with access to **specialist clinical assessment** and **ultrasound scanning**.

Pregnancy of Unknown Location (PUL)

1. **Diagnostic Criteria**:
   - **Positive pregnancy test**, but **no pregnancy visible on the scan**.
   - A pregnancy is considered ectopic until its location is confirmed.

2. **hCG Discriminatory Zones**:
   - For **transvaginal ultrasound**, consider a scan if **serum hCG is ≥ 1500 IU/l**.
   - For **abdominal ultrasonography**, consider a scan if **serum hCG is ≥ 6000 mIU/mL**.

3. **Diagnostic Approach**:
   - Do **not** use serum hCG or progesterone levels alone to determine the pregnancy's location.
   - Prioritize **clinical symptoms** over serum hCG levels in women with PUL.
   - Continuously review the woman's condition if symptoms change, regardless of previous assessments.

4. **Management**:
    - If a viable intrauterine pregnancy is confirmed, refer to **antenatal care (ANC)**.
    - If a viable intrauterine pregnancy is not confirmed, refer for **immediate clinical review by a senior gynaecologist**.
    - Inform the woman if the pregnancy is unlikely to continue, but this cannot be confirmed immediately. Provide both **oral and written information**.
    - Advise her to take a **urine pregnancy test 14 days** after the second serum hCG test:
        - If **negative**, no further action is needed.
        - If **positive**, she should return for a clinical review within **24 hours**.

5. **Follow-Up and Risk Assessment**:
    - For low-risk cases (failing PUL or viable intrauterine pregnancy), regular follow-up may be sufficient.
    - For high-risk cases (suspected ectopic pregnancy), immediate attention and possible intervention are required.

Single Best Answer (SBA) Questions

SBA 1

Question: Which of the following is the most appropriate action when a woman presents with vaginal bleeding and a positive pregnancy test, but no pregnancy is visible on the ultrasound scan?
a) Immediate surgical intervention
b) Reassure and discharge
c) Repeat serum hCG in 48 hours
d) Start progesterone therapy
e) Perform a diagnostic laparoscopy

SBA 2

Question: What is the earliest gestational age at which an early pregnancy assessment service should be available?
a) 4 weeks
b) 5 weeks
c) 6 weeks
d) 7 weeks
e) 8 weeks

SBA 3

Question: What is the key feature of a pregnancy of unknown location (PUL)?

a) Positive pregnancy test with visible intrauterine sac
b) Positive pregnancy test but no pregnancy visible on

scan
c) Negative pregnancy test with visible intrauterine sac
d) Negative pregnancy test with no pregnancy visible on scan
e) Pregnancy symptoms without a positive test or visible sac

SBA 4

Question: At what serum hCG level should a transvaginal ultrasound be considered in a woman with a positive pregnancy test but no visible pregnancy on the scan?
a) 1000 IU/l
b) 1500 IU/l
c) 2000 IU/l
d) 2500 IU/l
e) 3000 IU/l

SBA 5

Question: What is the primary goal of an early pregnancy assessment service?
a) To provide routine antenatal care
b) To manage complications in late pregnancy
c) To assess and manage early pregnancy complications
d) To provide postnatal care
e) To offer fertility treatments

SBA 6

Question: If an early pregnancy assessment service is unavailable, where should a woman with severe abdominal pain and a positive pregnancy test be referred?
a) General Practitioner (GP)
b) Accident & Emergency (A&E) department
c) Maternity ward
d) Fertility clinic
e) Outpatient clinic

SBA 7

Question: Which group of women is allowed to self-refer to an early pregnancy assessment service?
a) Women with no previous pregnancy history
b) Women with a history of recurrent miscarriage, previous ectopic pregnancy, or molar pregnancy
c) All pregnant women
d) Women over 40 years old
e) Women with a history of preterm labour

SBA 8

Question: What should be the next step for a woman with PUL and worsening abdominal pain, despite normal initial assessments?
a) Discharge with reassurance
b) Repeat serum hCG in 2 weeks
c) Immediate clinical review by a senior gynaecologist
d) Perform a repeat ultrasound after 7 days
e) Advise bed rest and hydration

SBA 9

Question: When is it appropriate to advise a woman with a PUL to take a urine pregnancy test at home?
a) 3 days after the initial scan
b) 7 days after the initial scan
c) 10 days after the initial scan
d) 14 days after the second serum hCG test
e) 21 days after the second serum hCG test

SBA 10

Question: What is the recommended management for a woman with a confirmed viable intrauterine pregnancy after initial concerns about a PUL?
a) Immediate referral to surgery
b) Discharge with routine antenatal care
c) Start high-dose progesterone therapy
d) Repeat hCG every 48 hours
e) Weekly ultrasound scans until 20 weeks

SBA 11

Question: In a woman with PUL, what should be prioritized in her assessment?
a) Serum hCG levels
b) Serum progesterone levels
c) Clinical symptoms
d) Fetal heart rate
e) Endometrial thickness on ultrasound

SBA 12

Question: What is the significance of a serum hCG level greater than 6000 mIU/mL in a woman undergoing abdominal ultrasonography?
a) Immediate surgery is required
b) A viable intrauterine pregnancy is confirmed
c) Ectopic pregnancy is excluded
d) A pregnancy should be visible on ultrasound
e) Pregnancy is unlikely to continue

SBA 13

Question: How soon should anti-D immunoglobulin be administered following a potentially sensitising event in a Rh D-negative woman?
a) Within 12 hours
b) Within 24 hours
c) Within 48 hours
d) Within 72 hours
e) Within 96 hours

SBA 14

Question: What is the appropriate follow-up for a woman with a PUL who has a negative urine pregnancy test 14 days after her second hCG test?
a) Perform an ultrasound scan
b) No further action needed
c) Repeat hCG levels
d) Refer to a fertility specialist
e) Advise admission to the hospital

SBA 15

Question: What is the first step in managing a woman with a PUL who presents with shoulder tip pain?
a) Repeat urine pregnancy test
b) Immediate clinical review for possible ectopic pregnancy
c) Start oral progesterone
d) Schedule a follow-up scan in one week
e) Discharge with bed rest advice

SBA 16

Question: For a woman with a history of recurrent miscarriage and a positive pregnancy test, what is the most appropriate initial referral?
a) Self-referral to early pregnancy assessment service
b) Referral to the general practitioner
c) Referral to a fertility clinic
d) Referral to the Accident & Emergency department
e) Referral to a midwife

SBA 17

Question: What is the recommended management for a Rh D-negative woman who experiences a first-trimester miscarriage at 8 weeks and does not undergo surgical management?
a) No anti-D immunoglobulin needed
b) Administer 250 IU anti-D immunoglobulin

c) Administer 500 IU anti-D immunoglobulin
d) Administer 1000 IU anti-D immunoglobulin
e) Perform a Kleihauer-Betke test first

SBA 18

Question: What is the most likely cause of a PUL when the initial hCG levels are stable and the woman is asymptomatic?
a) Intrauterine pregnancy
b) Ectopic pregnancy
c) Complete miscarriage
d) Failing pregnancy of unknown location
e) Molar pregnancy

SBA 19

Question: Which investigation is NOT routinely recommended for women with a pregnancy of unknown location?
a) Serum hCG levels
b) Serum progesterone levels
c) Ultrasound scan
d) Culdocentesis
e) Clinical symptom review

SBA 20

Question: What is the appropriate action for a woman with PUL who has an hCG level of 2000 IU/L, minimal symptoms, and no visible intrauterine pregnancy?
a) Discharge with reassurance
b) Repeat hCG in 48 hours
c) Perform an immediate laparoscopy

d) Start methotrexate therapy
e) Refer for a second opinion

Extended Match Questions (EMQ)

EMQ 1: Diagnostic Approach in Pregnancy of Unknown Location (PUL)

Lead-in Statement:
For each of the following clinical presentations, select the most appropriate diagnostic action from the list below.

Options:
A) Immediate transvaginal ultrasound
B) Serial serum hCG measurements
C) Expectant management
D) Laparoscopy
E) Serum progesterone measurement

Scenarios:

1. A 28-year-old woman presents with 5 weeks of amenorrhea, mild spotting, and a serum hCG level of 1300 IU/L. No gestational sac is visible on transvaginal ultrasound.

2. A 32-year-old woman has 6 weeks of amenorrhea and mild lower abdominal pain. Her serum hCG level is 1000 IU/L, and no pregnancy is visible on transvaginal ultrasound.

3. A 29-year-old woman with 7 weeks of amenorrhea presents with moderate abdominal pain and a serum hCG level of 2000 IU/L. Transvaginal ultrasound shows no intrauterine pregnancy, but free fluid is noted in the pelvis.

4. A 30-year-old woman with a positive pregnancy test presents with light spotting and a serum hCG level of 1500 IU/L. Transvaginal ultrasound does not show a pregnancy.

5. A 34-year-old woman presents with 4 weeks of amenorrhea and minimal symptoms. Her serum hCG level is 800 IU/L, and no gestational sac is seen on transvaginal ultrasound.

EMQ 2: Management of Ectopic Pregnancy in the Context of PUL

Lead-in Statement:
For each of the following clinical scenarios, select the most appropriate management option from the list below.

Options:
A) Methotrexate therapy
B) Laparoscopic salpingectomy
C) Expectant management
D) Repeat serum hCG in 48 hours
E) Immediate surgical intervention

Scenarios:

1. A 27-year-old woman with 8 weeks of amenorrhea presents with moderate abdominal pain and a serum hCG level of 2500 IU/L. Transvaginal ultrasound shows no intrauterine pregnancy but reveals free fluid in the pelvis.

2. A 26-year-old woman with 6 weeks of amenorrhea presents with mild abdominal pain and a serum hCG level of 1000 IU/L. No intrauterine pregnancy is seen on ultrasound.

3. A 30-year-old woman with a previous ectopic pregnancy presents with 5 weeks of amenorrhea, mild vaginal bleeding, and a serum hCG level of

2000 IU/L. Ultrasound does not show an intrauterine pregnancy.

4. A 29-year-old woman with 7 weeks of amenorrhea presents with severe abdominal pain and a serum hCG level of 5000 IU/L. Ultrasound shows a large amount of free fluid in the pelvis and no intrauterine pregnancy.

5. A 31-year-old woman with 6 weeks of amenorrhea and mild symptoms has a serum hCG level of 1200 IU/L and no visible pregnancy on ultrasound. She prefers to avoid surgical intervention.

EMQ 3: Referral and Follow-up in Early Pregnancy Assessment Services

Lead-in Statement:
For each of the following clinical scenarios, select the most appropriate referral or follow-up action from the list below.

Options:
A) Immediate referral to a senior gynaecologist
B) Follow-up scan in 7 days
C) Urgent referral to early pregnancy assessment service
D) Routine antenatal care
E) No further action needed

Scenarios:
1. A 28-year-old woman presents with 6 weeks of amenorrhea and mild vaginal bleeding.

Transvaginal ultrasound confirms a viable intrauterine pregnancy.

2. A 32-year-old woman with 8 weeks of amenorrhea presents with severe pelvic pain and a serum hCG level of 6000 IU/L. No pregnancy is seen on transvaginal ultrasound.

3. A 26-year-old woman presents with 5 weeks of amenorrhea and light spotting. Serum hCG is 1500 IU/L, and ultrasound shows no intrauterine pregnancy.

4. A 35-year-old woman with a history of recurrent miscarriages presents with 7 weeks of amenorrhea and spotting. Transvaginal ultrasound shows a gestational sac but no fetal heartbeat.

5. A 29-year-old woman presents with 7 weeks of amenorrhea and a positive pregnancy test. Ultrasound reveals an intrauterine pregnancy with a fetal heartbeat.

EMQ 4: Criteria for Self-Referral to Early Pregnancy Assessment Services

Lead-in Statement:
For each of the following scenarios, select the most appropriate criteria for self-referral from the list below.

Options:
A) Previous ectopic pregnancy
B) Recurrent miscarriage
C) History of molar pregnancy
D) No self-referral, requires professional assessment first
E) Severe abdominal pain

Scenarios:

1. A 30-year-old woman with two previous miscarriages at 9 and 10 weeks of gestation presents with 5 weeks of amenorrhea and mild spotting.
2. A 29-year-old woman with a history of molar pregnancy is now 7 weeks pregnant and is experiencing light vaginal bleeding.
3. A 32-year-old woman with a previous ectopic pregnancy presents with 6 weeks of amenorrhea and mild lower abdominal pain.
4. A 27-year-old woman with no significant medical history presents with 6 weeks of amenorrhea and moderate abdominal pain.
5. A 34-year-old woman with no history of ectopic pregnancy or recurrent miscarriage presents with 7 weeks of amenorrhea and spotting.

EMQ 5: Investigations for Suspected Ectopic Pregnancy

Lead-in Statement:
For each of the following clinical presentations, select the most appropriate investigation from the list below.

Options:
A) Transvaginal ultrasound
B) Serum hCG measurement
C) Serum progesterone measurement
D) Diagnostic laparoscopy
E) Abdominal ultrasound

Scenarios:
1. A 30-year-old woman presents with 7 weeks of amenorrhea, lower abdominal pain, and a serum hCG level of 1800 IU/L. No intrauterine

pregnancy is visible on the transvaginal ultrasound.

2. A 29-year-old woman with 6 weeks of amenorrhea presents with light vaginal bleeding and a serum hCG level of 900 IU/L. No gestational sac is seen on ultrasound.

3. A 28-year-old woman with 8 weeks of amenorrhea presents with moderate abdominal pain and a serum hCG level of 2500 IU/L. Transvaginal ultrasound shows no intrauterine pregnancy and moderate free fluid in the pelvis.

4. A 32-year-old woman with 7 weeks of amenorrhea presents with sudden onset severe abdominal pain. Ultrasound is inconclusive.

5. A 35-year-old woman with a history of ectopic pregnancy presents with 6 weeks of amenorrhea and mild lower abdominal pain. Serum hCG level is 1500 IU/L, and no intrauterine pregnancy is seen on ultrasound.

EMQ 6: Referral Criteria to Early Pregnancy Assessment Services (EPAS)

Lead-in Statement:
For each of the following scenarios, select the most appropriate referral criteria from the list below.

Options:
A) History of ectopic pregnancy
B) Severe abdominal pain
C) Recurrent miscarriage
D) Professional assessment required before referral
E) History of molar pregnancy

Scenarios:

1. A 31-year-old woman presents with 7 weeks of amenorrhea, mild spotting, and a history of a previous ectopic pregnancy.

2. A 28-year-old woman with 6 weeks of amenorrhea and a history of two consecutive miscarriages presents with light bleeding.

3. A 32-year-old woman with 7 weeks of amenorrhea and a history of a molar pregnancy presents with light spotting.

4. A 29-year-old woman presents with 6 weeks of amenorrhea, moderate abdominal pain, and no previous history of ectopic pregnancy.

5. A 30-year-old woman with a history of uncomplicated pregnancies presents with 5 weeks of amenorrhea and mild discomfort.

EMQ 7: Initial Management of Pregnancy of Unknown Location (PUL)

Lead-in Statement:
For each of the following clinical scenarios, select the most appropriate initial management option from the list below.

Options:
A) Serial serum hCG measurement
B) Immediate transvaginal ultrasound
C) Expectant management
D) Methotrexate treatment
E) Diagnostic laparoscopy

Scenarios:

1. A 30-year-old woman presents with 6 weeks of amenorrhea, mild lower abdominal pain, and a serum

hCG level of 1200 IU/L. No gestational sac is seen on the initial transvaginal ultrasound.

2. A 32-year-old woman with 5 weeks of amenorrhea presents with mild vaginal spotting. Her serum hCG level is 1600 IU/L, and the transvaginal ultrasound shows no intrauterine pregnancy.

3. A 29-year-old woman with 7 weeks of amenorrhea presents with moderate lower abdominal pain and a serum hCG level of 3000 IU/L. Transvaginal ultrasound reveals free fluid in the pelvis.

4. A 27-year-old woman presents with 8 weeks of amenorrhea and severe abdominal pain. Her serum hCG level is 7000 IU/L, and the transvaginal ultrasound shows no intrauterine pregnancy.

5. A 31-year-old woman presents with 4 weeks of amenorrhea and minimal symptoms. Her serum hCG level is 600 IU/L, and no gestational sac is seen on ultrasound.

EMQ 8: Risk Factors for Ectopic Pregnancy

Lead-in Statement:
For each of the following scenarios, select the most appropriate risk factor from the list below.

Options:
A) Previous ectopic pregnancy
B) Tubal surgery
C) Pelvic inflammatory disease (PID)
D) Use of intrauterine contraceptive device (IUCD)
E) Previous molar pregnancy

Scenarios:

1. A 29-year-old woman with a history of PID presents with 6 weeks of amenorrhea and lower abdominal pain.

2. A 32-year-old woman with a history of tubal surgery presents with 5 weeks of amenorrhea and spotting.

3. A 30-year-old woman with a previous ectopic pregnancy presents with 7 weeks of amenorrhea and mild pelvic pain.

4. A 27-year-old woman who is using an IUCD presents with 8 weeks of amenorrhea and light bleeding.

5. A 28-year-old woman with a history of a molar pregnancy presents with 7 weeks of amenorrhea and lower abdominal discomfort.

EMQ 9: Follow-up in Early Pregnancy Assessment Services

Lead-in Statement:
For each of the following clinical presentations, select the most appropriate follow-up action from the list below.

Options:
A) Immediate referral to senior gynaecologist
B) Repeat serum hCG in 48 hours
C) Follow-up scan in 7 days
D) Routine antenatal care
E) Discharge with no further follow-up needed

Scenarios:

1. A 28-year-old woman presents with 6 weeks of amenorrhea and mild spotting. Transvaginal ultrasound confirms a viable intrauterine pregnancy with a fetal heartbeat.

2. A 32-year-old woman with 7 weeks of amenorrhea presents with severe pelvic pain. Her serum hCG level is 7000 IU/L, and no pregnancy is seen on transvaginal ultrasound.

3. A 29-year-old woman presents with 5 weeks of amenorrhea and light bleeding. Serum hCG is 1500 IU/L, and no gestational sac is seen on ultrasound.

4. A 34-year-old woman with a history of recurrent miscarriages presents with 7 weeks of amenorrhea. Ultrasound shows a gestational sac but no fetal heartbeat.

5. A 30-year-old woman with 8 weeks of amenorrhea presents with severe abdominal pain. Ultrasound reveals no intrauterine pregnancy, and free fluid is noted in the pelvis.

EMQ 10: Interpretation of Serum hCG Levels in PUL

Lead-in Statement:
For each of the following clinical scenarios, select the most appropriate interpretation or action based on the serum hCG levels from the list below.

Options:
A) Viable intrauterine pregnancy likely
B) Ectopic pregnancy likely
C) Pregnancy failing (PUL)
D) Repeat hCG in 48 hours
E) Ectopic pregnancy unlikely

Scenarios:

1. A 30-year-old woman with 6 weeks of amenorrhea has a serum hCG level of 1300 IU/L. No gestational sac is visible on transvaginal ultrasound.

2. A 32-year-old woman with 7 weeks of amenorrhea presents with a serum hCG level of 2500 IU/L. No intrauterine pregnancy is seen on ultrasound.

3. A 29-year-old woman presents with 5 weeks of amenorrhea and light bleeding. Her serum hCG level is 200 IU/L.

4. A 27-year-old woman with 8 weeks of amenorrhea has a serum hCG level of 5000 IU/L. No intrauterine pregnancy is visible on ultrasound, and free fluid is noted in the pelvis.

5. A 31-year-old woman with a previous ectopic pregnancy has a serum hCG level of 600 IU/L and no visible gestational sac on ultrasound.

Ectopic Pregnancy: A Comprehensive Overview

Definition and Incidence

- **Ectopic pregnancy** is the implantation of a fertilized egg outside the endometrial cavity, most commonly in the fallopian tube (about 95% of cases). Rarely, it can occur in the cervix, ovary, or abdominal cavity.
- **Incidence**: In the UK, it occurs in approximately 11 per 1000 pregnancies. Among women attending early pregnancy units, the incidence is about 2–3%.

Common Symptoms

- Abdominal or pelvic pain
- Amenorrhoea (missed period)
- Vaginal bleeding (with or without clots)
- Gastrointestinal symptoms
- Dizziness, fainting, or syncope
- Shoulder tip pain
- Urinary symptoms
- Passage of tissue
- Rectal pressure or pain on defecation

Common Signs

- Pelvic tenderness

- Adnexal tenderness
- Abdominal tenderness

Risk Factors

- Tubal surgery
- Pelvic inflammatory disease (PID)
- Smoking
- In vitro fertilization (IVF)
- It is important to note that about **one-third of women with an ectopic pregnancy have no known risk factors.**

Sites of Implantation

- **Fimbriae end**: 5%.
- **Ampullary section**: 80%
- **Isthmus**: 12%
- **Interstitial part of the tube**

Diagnostic Approach

- **Transvaginal ultrasound** is the diagnostic tool of choice for detecting tubal ectopic pregnancies.
    - **Findings**:
        - Homogeneous or non-cystic adnexal mass (50–60% of cases)
        - Empty extrauterine gestational sac (20–40%)
        - Extrauterine gestational sac containing a yolk sac and/or embryonic pole (15–20%)

- - The presence of an **adnexal mass** moving separately from the ovary and with an empty gestational sac, or complex inhomogeneous adnexal mass, is indicative of a tubal ectopic pregnancy.
- **Laparoscopy** is no longer the gold standard for diagnosis.

Management Options

Expectant Management

- For women with a pregnancy of less than 6 weeks' gestation who are bleeding but not in pain and have no risk factors.
  - **Instructions**:
    - Return if bleeding continues or pain develops.
    - Repeat urine pregnancy test after 7–10 days; if positive, further assessment is needed.

Methotrexate

- Suitable for women who are:
  - Hemodynamically stable.
  - Have low serum b-hCG (ideally <1500 IU/L, but can be up to 5000 IU/L).
  - Have an unruptured ectopic pregnancy with a mass smaller than 35 mm.
- **Success Rates**: 65–95% for single-dose methotrexate.
- **Adverse Effects**:

- o Common: Excessive flatulence and bloating.
- o Rare: Marrow suppression, pulmonary fibrosis, nonspecific pneumonitis, liver cirrhosis, renal failure, and gastric ulceration.
- Women treated with methotrexate should avoid conception for at least 3 months.

Surgical Management

- **Salpingectomy**: Recommended when the contralateral tube is healthy.
- **Salpingotomy**: Considered in women with fertility-reducing factors or only one tube.
  - o **Risks**: Up to 20% of women may require further treatment due to persistent trophoblast.
- **Laparotomy**: Reserved for hemodynamically unstable patients.

Follow-up Protocol

- **Post-salpingotomy**: Weekly serum b-hCG levels until less than 20 IU/L.
- **Post-salpingectomy**: Urine pregnancy test 3 weeks after surgery, with a follow-up if positive.

Special Cases

- **Interstitial Pregnancy**: Diagnosed via transvaginal ultrasound or MRI, with management options including methotrexate or surgical intervention (e.g., cornual resection).

Cervical Ectopic Pregnancy

- **Prevalence and Identification**: Cervical ectopic pregnancies are very rare, constituting less than 1% of all ectopic gestations. Diagnosis is based on specific ultrasound findings:
    - An empty uterine cavity.
    - A barrel-shaped cervix.
    - A gestational sac located below the internal cervical os.
    - Absence of the "sliding sign," where in a miscarriage, the gestational sac moves against the cervical canal with probe pressure, but in a cervical pregnancy, it does not.
    - Blood flow around the gestational sac on colour Doppler (not just fluid or blood in the cervix).
- **Management**:
    - **Medical Treatment**: Systemic methotrexate is effective, with an estimated success rate of approximately 91%. However, treatment is less effective with higher b-hCG levels (>10,000 IU), advanced gestational age (>9 weeks),

larger crown-rump length (>10 mm), or fetal cardiac activity.
- **Combination Therapy**: Combining systemic methotrexate with intra-amniotic injection may improve treatment success.
- **Surgical Treatment**: Reserved for severe cases with life-threatening bleeding due to high failure rates of surgical methods.

Heterotopic Pregnancy

- **Prevalence**: Heterotopic pregnancy, where both an intrauterine and ectopic pregnancy coexist, occurs in approximately 1 in 8,000 to 30,000 spontaneous conceptions, and up to 1% in assisted reproductive technology cases, especially with multiple embryo transfers.
- **Diagnosis**: A high index of suspicion is needed. Serum b-hCG levels are not very helpful in diagnosing heterotopic pregnancies.
- **Management**:
  - **Medical Management**: Methotrexate should only be used if the intrauterine pregnancy is nonviable or if the patient does not wish to continue with the pregnancy.
  - **Local Treatments**: Options include local injection of potassium chloride or hyperosmolar glucose combined with aspiration of the sac contents for stable women.

- **Surgical Treatment**: Preferred for women who are hemodynamically unstable and also an option for stable women.
- **Expectant Management**: Suitable if the ectopic pregnancy is nonviable based on ultrasound findings.

Caesarean Section Scar Ectopic Pregnancy (CSP) Summary

Incidence and Risk Factors:

- CSP occurs in 1 in 1800–2200 pregnancies.
- About 19% of women with a prior caesarean section (CS) will have a defect in the anterior myometrium at the CS scar level.
- Major risks include uterine rupture, haemorrhage, and hysterectomy.
- The recurrence risk is reported as 3.2–5.0%. Women with a CS for breech presentation may be at higher risk due to a poorly formed lower uterine segment.

Types of CSP:

- **Type 1 (Endogenic CSP):** Gestational sac implants on the scar and grows towards the uterine cavity.
- **Type 2 (Exogenic CSP):** Gestational sac is embedded in the scar and grows towards the bladder, with a thinner myometrial layer between

the sac and bladder, increasing the risk of rupture.

Ultrasound Diagnosis:

- **Criteria:**
    - Empty uterine cavity and closed cervical canal.
    - Gestational sac/placenta embedded in the previous CS scar.
    - Triangular/round or oval-shaped sac filling the scar niche.
    - Thin or absent myometrial layer between sac and bladder.
    - Potential presence of yolk sac, embryo, and cardiac activity.
    - Evidence of functional placental circulation on Doppler ultrasound.
    - Negative 'sliding sign' distinguishing from cervical miscarriage.
- **Imaging Techniques:**
    - Combined transabdominal and transvaginal ultrasound is preferred for high accuracy.
    - 3D ultrasound may complement 2D findings if needed.
    - MRI is useful for diagnosis, especially in later gestation or uncertain cases.

Management Options:

- **Expectant Management:** Rarely used, only in select cases.
- **Medical Management:**

- **Systemic Methotrexate:** Effective in cases with hCG levels <5000 IU/L and gestational age <8 weeks.
- **Local Injection and Embolization:** Includes methotrexate with sac aspiration, embryocides like potassium chloride or hyperosmolar glucose, and uterine artery chemoembolization.

- **Surgical Management:**
  - Options include dilation and surgical evacuation, hysteroscopic resection, various excision techniques (vaginal, laparoscopic, or open), and hysterectomy.
- **Combined or Sequential Management:**
  - Uterine artery embolization or chemoembolization followed by surgical evacuation or resection.
  - Methotrexate followed by surgical resection after an interval.

Specific Techniques:

- **In Lower-Segment CSP:** Suction evacuation of retained products under ultrasound guidance is common. A Schirodkar suture may be used to control bleeding post-evacuation.

Single Best Answer (SBA) Questions

SBA 21

A 28-year-old woman presents with sudden onset of lower abdominal pain and vaginal bleeding. She has a history of pelvic inflammatory disease and is sexually active. On examination, she is pale with a blood pressure of 90/60 mmHg and pulse of 110 bpm. A pelvic ultrasound shows free fluid in the pelvis, but no intrauterine pregnancy is visualised. What is the most likely diagnosis?

a) Threatened miscarriage
b) Ovarian torsion
c) Ectopic pregnancy
d) Endometriosis
e) Ruptured corpus luteum cyst

SBA 22

A 32-year-old woman presents with 6 weeks of amenorrhoea and left-sided pelvic pain. A urine pregnancy test is positive. Transvaginal ultrasound shows an adnexal mass with no intrauterine pregnancy. Her serum hCG level is 3000 IU/L. What is the next best step in management?

a) Laparoscopy
b) Expectant management
c) Methotrexate therapy
d) Dilation and curettage
e) Repeat ultrasound in one week

SBA 23

A 25-year-old woman with a history of tubal surgery presents with vaginal spotting and mild pelvic pain. She has a positive pregnancy test but her serum hCG level is 900 IU/L. A transvaginal ultrasound shows no intrauterine pregnancy and an adnexal mass is noted. What is the most appropriate management?

a) Surgical management
b) Methotrexate therapy
c) Expectant management
d) Laparoscopy
e) Hysteroscopy

SBA 24

A 30-year-old woman presents with amenorrhoea for 7 weeks and lower abdominal pain. She recently underwent IVF treatment. On ultrasound, there is an intrauterine pregnancy and a complex mass in the right adnexa. What is the most likely diagnosis?

a) Ovarian cyst
b) Pelvic inflammatory disease
c) Ectopic pregnancy
d) Heterotopic pregnancy
e) Corpus luteum cyst

SBA 25

A 34-year-old woman presents with severe abdominal pain and dizziness. She has a history of a prior ectopic pregnancy. Her blood pressure is 80/50 mmHg, and her pulse is 120 bpm. A pelvic ultrasound shows a large amount of free fluid in the pelvis. What is the most appropriate management?

a) Methotrexate therapy
b) Expectant management
c) Laparoscopy
d) Laparotomy
e) Intravenous fluids and observation

SBA 26

A 24-year-old woman presents with 5 weeks of amenorrhoea and right lower quadrant pain. Her serum hCG level is 1500 IU/L. A transvaginal ultrasound does not show any intrauterine or extrauterine pregnancy. What is the next best step?

a) Immediate laparoscopy
b) Expectant management
c) Repeat serum hCG in 48 hours
d) Methotrexate therapy
e) MRI of the pelvis

SBA 27

A 29-year-old woman presents with 8 weeks of amenorrhoea, lower abdominal pain, and vaginal bleeding. Her serum hCG level is 2500 IU/L. A transvaginal ultrasound reveals an adnexal mass with no intrauterine pregnancy. What is the most appropriate treatment?

a) Expectant management
b) Methotrexate therapy
c) Laparoscopy
d) Hysteroscopy
e) Medical termination of pregnancy

SBA 28

A 35-year-old woman presents with a 6-week history of amenorrhoea and lower abdominal pain. She has a serum hCG level of 4000 IU/L and an adnexal mass is found on transvaginal ultrasound, with no evidence of intrauterine pregnancy. What is the most likely diagnosis?

a) Ovarian cyst
b) Tubal pregnancy
c) Miscarriage
d) Fibroid
e) Endometriosis

SBA 29

A 27-year-old woman presents with a 7-week history of amenorrhoea, sharp lower abdominal pain, and shoulder tip pain. She has a positive pregnancy test, but ultrasound does not show an intrauterine pregnancy. What is the most likely diagnosis?

a) Miscarriage
b) Ovarian cyst rupture
c) Ectopic pregnancy
d) Appendicitis
e) Endometriosis

SBA 30

A 33-year-old woman presents to A&E with severe lower abdominal pain, dizziness, and a history of 6 weeks of amenorrhoea. Her vital signs are unstable, with a blood pressure of 85/55 mmHg and a pulse of 125 bpm. A pelvic ultrasound reveals significant free fluid in the abdomen. What is the next step in management?

a) Methotrexate therapy
b) Laparotomy
c) Laparoscopy
d) Expectant management
e) Hysteroscopy

SBA 31

A 23-year-old woman presents with amenorrhoea for 5 weeks and mild pelvic discomfort. A transvaginal ultrasound fails to demonstrate an intrauterine pregnancy, and her serum hCG level is 1200 IU/L. What is the most likely diagnosis?

a) Complete miscarriage
b) Early intrauterine pregnancy
c) Ectopic pregnancy
d) Pregnancy of unknown location
e) Ovarian cyst

SBA 32

A 26-year-old woman presents with 6 weeks of amenorrhoea, lower abdominal pain, and spotting. Her serum hCG level is 1400 IU/L, and a transvaginal ultrasound does not reveal an intrauterine pregnancy. What is the next best step?

a) Immediate laparoscopy
b) Expectant management
c) Repeat serum hCG in 48 hours
d) Methotrexate therapy
e) Dilation and curettage

SBA 33

A 29-year-old woman presents with sudden onset of severe lower abdominal pain and vaginal bleeding. She is hypotensive with a blood pressure of 90/60 mmHg and a pulse of 110 bpm. A transvaginal ultrasound shows a large amount of free fluid in the pelvis. What is the most likely diagnosis?

a) Miscarriage
b) Ovarian torsion
c) Ruptured ectopic pregnancy
d) Endometriosis
e) Appendicitis

SBA 34

A 24-year-old woman presents with 7 weeks of amenorrhoea, mild pelvic pain, and spotting. Her serum hCG level is 3000 IU/L, and a transvaginal ultrasound reveals an adnexal mass with no intrauterine pregnancy. She is haemodynamically stable. What is the most appropriate treatment?

a) Expectant management
b) Methotrexate therapy
c) Laparoscopy
d) Dilation and curettage
e) Medical termination of pregnancy

SBA 35

A 31-year-old woman presents with 8 weeks of amenorrhoea, lower abdominal pain, and vaginal bleeding. Her serum hCG level is 5000 IU/L. A transvaginal ultrasound reveals an adnexal mass with no intrauterine pregnancy. What is the next step in management?

a) Expectant management
b) Methotrexate therapy
c) Laparoscopy
d) Hysteroscopy
e) Medical termination of pregnancy

SBA 36

A 28-year-old woman presents with a history of pelvic inflammatory disease and a positive pregnancy test. She complains of lower abdominal pain and spotting. A transvaginal ultrasound shows an adnexal mass but no intrauterine pregnancy. What is the most likely diagnosis?

a) Miscarriage
b) Ectopic pregnancy
c) Ovarian cyst
d) Endometriosis
e) Appendicitis

SBA 37

A 27-year-old woman presents with amenorrhoea for 6 weeks, mild pelvic pain, and spotting. Her serum hCG level is 1800 IU/L. A transvaginal ultrasound shows a complex adnexal mass but no intrauterine pregnancy.

She is haemodynamically stable. What is the most appropriate treatment?

a) Expectant management
b) Methotrexate therapy
c) Laparoscopy
d) Dilation and curettage
e) Medical termination of pregnancy

SBA 38

A 30-year-old woman presents with lower abdominal pain, 7 weeks of amenorrhoea, and vaginal bleeding. An ultrasound scan shows a gestational sac in the right adnexa but no intrauterine pregnancy. What is the most likely diagnosis?

a) Ovarian cyst
b) Tubal pregnancy
c) Miscarriage
d) Fibroid
e) Endometriosis

SBA 39

A 35-year-old woman presents to A&E with severe abdominal pain and dizziness. She has a history of a previous ectopic pregnancy. Her vital signs are unstable. A pelvic ultrasound reveals a large amount of free fluid in the abdomen. What is the next step in management?

a) Methotrexate therapy
b) Laparotomy
c) Laparoscopy
d) Expectant management
e) Medical termination of pregnancy

SBA 40

A 32-year-old woman presents with 6 weeks of amenorrhoea, lower abdominal pain, and vaginal spotting. Her serum hCG level is 4000 IU/L, and a transvaginal ultrasound shows an adnexal mass but no intrauterine pregnancy. What is the most likely diagnosis?

a) Miscarriage
b) Ovarian cyst
c) Ectopic pregnancy

SBA 41

A 25-year-old woman presents with right lower abdominal pain and vaginal spotting. She has a history of pelvic inflammatory disease and is currently 7 weeks pregnant based on her last menstrual period. Ultrasound shows no intrauterine pregnancy but reveals an adnexal mass. What is the most likely diagnosis?

a) Ovarian cyst
b) Missed miscarriage
c) Ectopic pregnancy
d) Appendicitis
e) Normal intrauterine pregnancy

SBA 42

A 33-year-old woman, who recently underwent IVF, presents with severe lower abdominal pain and fainting. Her vital signs show hypotension and tachycardia. Transvaginal ultrasound reveals an intrauterine gestation and an adnexal mass with free fluid in the pelvis. What is the most appropriate next step?

a) Expectant management
b) Methotrexate therapy
c) Diagnostic laparoscopy

d) Emergency laparotomy
e) Pelvic MRI

SBA 43
A 29-year-old woman presents with shoulder tip pain, vaginal bleeding, and a positive pregnancy test. Her hCG level is 2000 IU/L, and ultrasound shows no intrauterine pregnancy. What is the most likely cause of her symptoms?
a) Threatened miscarriage
b) Normal intrauterine pregnancy
c) Ectopic pregnancy
d) Ovarian torsion
e) Endometriosis

SBA 44
A 31-year-old woman presents with amenorrhoea, vaginal spotting, and a serum hCG of 500 IU/L. Transvaginal ultrasound is inconclusive. What is the best next step in management?
a) Emergency laparotomy
b) Repeat hCG in 48 hours
c) Methotrexate therapy
d) Diagnostic laparoscopy
e) Expectant management

SBA 45
A 34-year-old woman with a history of tubal surgery presents with severe left lower abdominal pain and fainting. Her hCG level is 3000 IU/L, and ultrasound shows a left adnexal mass with free fluid. What is the most appropriate management?
a) Expectant management
b) Methotrexate therapy

c) Salpingotomy
d) Laparoscopy
e) Emergency laparotomy

SBA 46
A 26-year-old woman at 6 weeks' gestation presents with mild abdominal pain and vaginal spotting. Her hCG level is 1000 IU/L. Transvaginal ultrasound shows no intrauterine pregnancy and a small right adnexal mass. She is hemodynamically stable. What is the best management approach?
a) Expectant management
b) Methotrexate therapy
c) Emergency laparotomy
d) Laparoscopy
e) Pelvic MRI

SBA 47
A 30-year-old woman presents with sudden severe abdominal pain, dizziness, and vaginal bleeding at 8 weeks' gestation. Her blood pressure is 80/50 mmHg, and ultrasound shows an empty uterus and free fluid in the abdomen. What is the most likely diagnosis?
a) Ruptured ovarian cyst
b) Acute appendicitis
c) Ruptured ectopic pregnancy
d) Miscarriage
e) Ovarian torsion

SBA 48
A 27-year-old woman with a positive pregnancy test presents with intermittent spotting and right-sided pelvic pain. Her hCG level is 1200 IU/L. Ultrasound shows no intrauterine pregnancy and an 8 mm adnexal mass. She

is stable with no significant free fluid. What is the most appropriate treatment?
a) Expectant management
b) Methotrexate therapy
c) Emergency laparotomy
d) Laparoscopy
e) Salpingectomy

SBA 49
A 35-year-old woman presents with a history of amenorrhoea, abdominal pain, and spotting. Her hCG level is 8000 IU/L. Ultrasound shows an empty uterus with a 3 cm adnexal mass. What is the best next step in management?
a) Repeat hCG in 48 hours
b) Methotrexate therapy
c) Expectant management
d) Laparoscopy
e) Laparotomy

SBA 50
A 28-year-old woman, 7 weeks pregnant, presents with left lower abdominal pain and vaginal bleeding. Her hCG level is 3000 IU/L. Ultrasound shows an empty uterus and a left adnexal mass. What is the most likely diagnosis?
a) Missed miscarriage
b) Ovarian cyst
c) Ectopic pregnancy
d) Normal intrauterine pregnancy
e) Ovarian torsion

SBA 51
A 30-year-old woman presents with amenorrhoea, left lower abdominal pain, and vaginal bleeding. Her serum β-hCG is 3000 IU/L. Transvaginal ultrasound reveals an empty uterus and a 2 cm left adnexal mass. What is the most likely diagnosis?
a) Ovarian cyst
b) Pelvic inflammatory disease
c) Ectopic pregnancy
d) Endometriosis
e) Normal intrauterine pregnancy

SBA 52
What percentage of ectopic pregnancies are located in the ampullary section of the fallopian tube?
a) 95%
b) 80%
c) 50%
d) 30%
e) 10%

SBA 53
A 32-year-old woman presents with severe pelvic pain, dizziness, and a positive pregnancy test. Her blood pressure is 90/60 mmHg, and ultrasound shows an empty uterus with free fluid in the abdomen. What is the most appropriate initial management?
a) Expectant management
b) Methotrexate therapy
c) Laparoscopy
d) Laparotomy
e) Pelvic MRI

SBA 54
Which of the following is a known risk factor for ectopic pregnancy?
a) Use of oral contraceptives
b) Previous Caesarean section
c) Pelvic inflammatory disease
d) Fibroids
e) Polycystic ovary syndrome

SBA 55
What is the approximate incidence of ectopic pregnancy in the UK per 1000 pregnancies?
a) 5
b) 11
c) 25
d) 50
e) 100

SBA 56
A 28-year-old woman with a history of infertility presents with severe right lower quadrant pain and vaginal bleeding. Her serum β-hCG is 1500 IU/L, and ultrasound shows a complex right adnexal mass. What is the most appropriate management?
a) Expectant management
b) Methotrexate therapy
c) Diagnostic laparoscopy
d) Pelvic MRI
e) Observation only

SBA 57
Which site is the least common location for ectopic pregnancies?
a) Ampullary section

b) Isthmus
c) Cervix
d) Ovary
e) Abdominal cavity

SBA 58
A 27-year-old woman at 6 weeks' gestation presents with spotting and right-sided abdominal pain. Her serum β-hCG is 1200 IU/L. Ultrasound shows an empty uterus and a right adnexal mass. She is haemodynamically stable. What is the most appropriate management?
a) Expectant management
b) Methotrexate therapy
c) Emergency laparotomy
d) Laparoscopy
e) Repeat ultrasound in 7 days

SBA 59
Which ultrasound finding is most indicative of a tubal ectopic pregnancy?
a) Homogeneous ovarian cyst
b) Empty intrauterine gestational sac
c) Extrauterine gestational sac with a yolk sac
d) Presence of ovarian cysts in both ovaries
e) Thickened endometrium

SBA 60
What is the success rate range for single-dose methotrexate in treating ectopic pregnancy?
a) 25–45%
b) 45–65%
c) 65–95%
d) 95–100%
e) 100%

SBA 61
A 33-year-old woman with a positive pregnancy test presents with severe lower abdominal pain and hypotension. Transvaginal ultrasound shows an empty uterus and free fluid in the abdomen. What is the most likely diagnosis?
a) Ruptured ectopic pregnancy
b) Ovarian torsion
c) Miscarriage
d) Endometriosis
e) Acute appendicitis

SBA 62
A 29-year-old woman with a previous history of ectopic pregnancy presents with amenorrhoea and mild abdominal pain. Her serum β-hCG is 4000 IU/L. Transvaginal ultrasound is inconclusive. What is the next best step?
a) Emergency laparotomy
b) Methotrexate therapy
c) Repeat β-hCG in 48 hours
d) Expectant management
e) Laparoscopy

SBA 63
What is the recurrence risk of ectopic pregnancy in women with a history of Caesarean section scar ectopic pregnancy?
a) 0.5–1.0%
b) 1.0–2.0%
c) 3.2–5.0%
d) 7.0–10.0%
e) 15–20%

SBA 64
A 34-year-old woman presents with abdominal pain and vaginal bleeding. Her serum β-hCG is 9000 IU/L. Transvaginal ultrasound reveals an empty uterus with a left adnexal mass. What is the most appropriate management?
a) Methotrexate therapy
b) Expectant management
c) Pelvic MRI
d) Laparoscopy
e) Laparotomy

SBA 65
What is the first-line treatment for a stable patient with an unruptured ectopic pregnancy, a mass less than 35 mm, and a β-hCG level of 2000 IU/L?
a) Emergency laparotomy
b) Salpingectomy
c) Methotrexate therapy
d) Expectant management
e) Laparoscopy

SBA 66
Which of the following sites of implantation is most common for an ectopic pregnancy?
a) Cervical
b) Ovarian
c) Abdominal cavity
d) Ampullary section of the fallopian tube
e) Isthmus of the fallopian tube

SBA 67
A 25-year-old woman with a history of PID presents with

sharp lower abdominal pain and vaginal spotting. Her serum β-hCG is 1800 IU/L. Ultrasound shows no intrauterine pregnancy. What is the most likely diagnosis?
a) Miscarriage
b) Ectopic pregnancy
c) Ovarian torsion
d) Endometriosis
e) Normal intrauterine pregnancy

SBA 68
Which of the following conditions is a contraindication for methotrexate therapy in the management of ectopic pregnancy?
a) Hemodynamically stable patient
b) Mass size of 25 mm
c) β-hCG level of 5000 IU/L
d) Desire for future fertility
e) Hemoperitoneum on ultrasound

SBA 69
A 31-year-old woman presents with right-sided pelvic pain and spotting. Her serum β-hCG is 2500 IU/L. Ultrasound reveals an adnexal mass with a yolk sac. She is stable. What is the most appropriate next step?
a) Expectant management
b) Methotrexate therapy
c) Laparotomy
d) Laparoscopy
e) Repeat ultrasound in 7 days

SBA 70
Which of the following is the least likely location for an ectopic pregnancy?

a) Ampullary section of the fallopian tube
b) Isthmus of the fallopian tube
c) Cervix
d) Ovary
e) Endometrial cavity

Extended Match Questions (EMQ)

EMQ 11

Theme: Risk Factors for Ectopic Pregnancy
Options:
a) Tubal surgery
b) Pelvic inflammatory disease (PID)
c) Smoking
d) In vitro fertilization (IVF)
e) No known risk factors

Scenarios:

1. A 28-year-old woman with a history of tubal ligation presents with abdominal pain and a positive pregnancy test.
2. A 35-year-old smoker presents with amenorrhoea and pelvic pain. Ultrasound confirms an ectopic pregnancy.
3. A 30-year-old woman who has undergone two cycles of IVF now presents with acute abdominal pain.
4. A 32-year-old woman with a history of chlamydia and PID presents with lower abdominal pain and spotting.
5. A 25-year-old woman with no significant medical history presents with lower abdominal pain and a positive pregnancy test.

EMQ 12

Theme: Sites of Ectopic Implantation
Options:
a) Ampullary section of the fallopian tube
b) Isthmic section of the fallopian tube

c) Fimbriae end of the fallopian tube
d) Interstitial part of the fallopian tube
e) Cervix

Scenarios:

1. A 27-year-old woman presents with severe lower abdominal pain. Ultrasound shows an ectopic pregnancy in the ampullary region.
2. A 30-year-old woman presents with vaginal bleeding and pain. Ultrasound reveals a pregnancy in the cervical region.
3. A 32-year-old woman with a positive pregnancy test presents with severe left-sided pain. Ultrasound confirms a fimbrial ectopic pregnancy.
4. A 28-year-old woman is found to have an ectopic pregnancy in the isthmic region of the fallopian tube during an exploratory laparoscopy.
5. A 35-year-old woman presents with shock and a history of amenorrhoea. Ultrasound suggests an interstitial ectopic pregnancy.

EMQ 13

Theme: Clinical Presentation of Ectopic Pregnancy
Options:
a) Abdominal or pelvic pain
b) Vaginal bleeding
c) Amenorrhoea
d) Shoulder tip pain
e) Syncope

Scenarios:

1. A 29-year-old woman presents with sudden, sharp left lower quadrant pain and a positive pregnancy test.

2. A 32-year-old woman reports 6 weeks of amenorrhoea, followed by the onset of vaginal bleeding.
3. A 25-year-old woman presents to A&E with dizziness, fainting, and lower abdominal pain. She is confirmed to be pregnant.
4. A 34-year-old woman complains of severe right-sided abdominal pain radiating to the shoulder tip. Ultrasound shows a ruptured ectopic pregnancy.
5. A 30-year-old woman presents with a history of amenorrhoea and pelvic pain, with associated vaginal bleeding.

EMQ 14

Theme: Diagnostic Ultrasound Findings in Ectopic Pregnancy
Options:
a) Empty uterus
b) Complex adnexal mass
c) Free fluid in the pelvis
d) Gestational sac with yolk sac in adnexa
e) Pseudogestational sac in the uterus

Scenarios:

1. A 27-year-old woman with a positive pregnancy test has an ultrasound showing an empty uterus and a complex adnexal mass.
2. A 29-year-old woman presents with amenorrhoea and spotting. Ultrasound shows a pseudogestational sac in the uterus but no intrauterine pregnancy.
3. A 35-year-old woman with lower abdominal pain undergoes ultrasound, which reveals a gestational sac with a yolk sac in the adnexa.

4. A 28-year-old woman presents with acute abdominal pain. Ultrasound shows free fluid in the pelvis and an empty uterus.
5. A 26-year-old woman presents with pelvic pain. Ultrasound reveals an empty uterus and a mass in the ampullary region.

EMQ 15

Theme: Management of Ectopic Pregnancy Based on Clinical Scenario
Options:
a) Methotrexate
b) Expectant management
c) Salpingectomy
d) Salpingotomy
e) Laparotomy

Scenarios:

1. A 28-year-old woman with a confirmed unruptured ectopic pregnancy, stable vitals, and a β-hCG level of 1200 IU/L.
2. A 32-year-old woman with a ruptured ectopic pregnancy and haemodynamic instability.
3. A 25-year-old woman with a small ectopic pregnancy, no symptoms, and declining β-hCG levels.
4. A 30-year-old woman with a viable contralateral tube and an ectopic pregnancy confirmed in the right fallopian tube.
5. A 35-year-old woman with only one fallopian tube, presenting with a confirmed ectopic pregnancy.

EMQ 16

Theme: Sites of Ectopic Implantation
Options:
a) Cervical
b) Ampullary
c) Isthmic
d) Fimbrial
e) Interstitial

Scenarios:

1. A 29-year-old woman presents with severe abdominal pain. Transvaginal ultrasound shows a gestational sac in the ampullary region of the fallopian tube.
2. A 34-year-old woman presents with heavy vaginal bleeding. Ultrasound reveals a gestational sac located in the cervix.
3. A 31-year-old woman with a history of PID presents with lower abdominal pain. Ultrasound shows an ectopic pregnancy in the isthmic part of the fallopian tube.
4. A 27-year-old woman with amenorrhoea and pain is found to have an ectopic pregnancy in the fimbrial end of the tube.
5. A 33-year-old woman with a positive pregnancy test and severe pelvic pain is diagnosed with an interstitial ectopic pregnancy.

EMQ 17

Theme: Risk Factors for Ectopic Pregnancy
Options:
a) Prior ectopic pregnancy
b) Intrauterine device (IUD) use
c) Tubal surgery
d) Pelvic inflammatory disease (PID)
e) No identifiable risk factor

Scenarios:

1. A 28-year-old woman with a history of a previous ectopic pregnancy now presents with abdominal pain and a positive pregnancy test.
2. A 30-year-old woman with a history of PID presents with lower abdominal pain and a positive pregnancy test.
3. A 32-year-old woman using an IUD presents with abdominal pain and a positive pregnancy test.
4. A 35-year-old woman with a history of tubal surgery presents with pelvic pain and a positive pregnancy test.
5. A 26-year-old woman with no known risk factors presents with pelvic pain and a positive pregnancy test.

EMQ 18

Theme: Follow-Up Management of Ectopic Pregnancy
Options:
a) Repeat β-hCG in 48 hours
b) Weekly β-hCG until <20 IU/L
c) Urine pregnancy test in 3 weeks
d) Immediate laparoscopy
e) MRI assessment

Scenarios:

1. A 28-year-old woman who underwent methotrexate treatment for ectopic pregnancy needs follow-up to confirm resolution.
2. A 32-year-old woman post-salpingectomy for a ruptured ectopic pregnancy requires further evaluation.
3. A 30-year-old woman with persistent abdominal pain following salpingotomy needs follow-up.

4. A 25-year-old woman with an interstitial ectopic pregnancy diagnosed by ultrasound is under observation.
5. A 29-year-old woman post-surgical management of a cervical ectopic pregnancy requires follow-up.

EMQ 19

Theme: Methotrexate Use in Ectopic Pregnancy
Options:
a) Hemodynamically stable with low β-hCG (<1500 IU/L)
b) Unruptured ectopic pregnancy with a mass smaller than 35 mm
c) High β-hCG (>5000 IU/L)
d) Presence of fetal cardiac activity
e) Tubal rupture with haemodynamic instability

Scenarios:

1. A 26-year-old woman with an unruptured ectopic pregnancy, β-hCG of 1300 IU/L, and stable vitals.
2. A 29-year-old woman with a small, unruptured ectopic pregnancy and a β-hCG of 4800 IU/L.
3. A 33-year-old woman with an ectopic pregnancy showing fetal cardiac activity.
4. A 31-year-old woman presenting with haemodynamic instability and a ruptured ectopic pregnancy.
5. A 28-year-old woman with a small ectopic mass of 30 mm, no symptoms, and a β-hCG level of 1600 IU/L.

EMQ 20

Theme: Cervical Ectopic Pregnancy Management
Options:

a) Systemic methotrexate
b) Intra-amniotic injection
c) Surgical management due to life-threatening bleeding
d) Expectant management
e) Methotrexate with intra-amniotic injection

Scenarios:

1. A 28-year-old woman diagnosed with a cervical ectopic pregnancy, β-hCG of 8000 IU/L, and no fetal cardiac activity.
2. A 31-year-old woman with a cervical ectopic pregnancy and significant vaginal bleeding.
3. A 34-year-old woman with a cervical ectopic pregnancy and fetal cardiac activity at 10 weeks

Early Pregnancy Ultrasound

- **Dating the Pregnancy:**
    - **Crown-Rump Length (CRL):** The most accurate method for determining gestational age up to 13+6 weeks. Measure the CRL in a true mid-sagittal plane with the genital tubercle and fetal spine longitudinally visible. The measurement should be the mean of three discrete CRL measurements.
    - **Head Circumference:** For foetuses with a CRL greater than 84 mm (around 14+0 weeks), head circumference becomes more accurate than CRL for dating.
    - **Mean Sac Diameter:** Not recommended for estimating the estimated due date (EDD) as it has less accuracy compared to CRL and head circumference.
- **Assessment of Viability:**
    - **Fetal Heartbeat:** If a fetal heartbeat is visible, this confirms viability. If not visible but a fetal pole is present, measure the CRL.
    - **No Visible Fetal Pole:** Use the mean gestational sac diameter measurement if the fetal pole is not visible.
- **Follow-Up and Reassessment:**
    - **CRL Measurement:** If CRL is less than 7.0 mm and there is no visible heartbeat on a vaginal ultrasound, a second scan should be performed at least 7 days later. If CRL is 7.0 mm or more without a visible heartbeat, seek a second opinion or follow up with a scan at least 7 days later.

- **Gestational Sac Diameter:** For a sac diameter less than 25.0 mm with no visible fetal pole, perform a second scan a minimum of 7 days later. For a sac diameter of 25.0 mm or more without a fetal pole, seek a second opinion or rescan after 7 days.
  - **No Visible Heartbeat or Fetal Pole:** When using transabdominal ultrasound, if there is no heartbeat or fetal pole, record the size and perform a follow-up scan at least 14 days later.
- **Menstrual Dates:**
  - **LMP-Based Dating:** Do not rely solely on LMP for gestational age due to variability. Adjust the EDD based on the earliest and most accurate ultrasound measurements if there is a discrepancy of more than 7 days.

2. Diagnosis of Miscarriage

- **Complete Miscarriage:**
  - **Diagnosis:** If there is no previous scan confirming an intrauterine pregnancy, consider the possibility of a pregnancy of unknown location. Advise follow-up (such as serial hCG levels or additional scans) until a definitive diagnosis is made.
- **Threatened Miscarriage:**
  - **Advice:** For women with vaginal bleeding but a confirmed intrauterine pregnancy and fetal heartbeat, advise them to return for further assessment if the bleeding worsens or persists beyond 14 days. If

bleeding resolves, they should proceed with routine antenatal care.

3. Miscarriage Management

- **Expectant Management:**
  - **First-Line Treatment:** This is usually the first approach as most women do not need further treatment. Provide oral and written information about other treatment options. Consider alternatives if there is a high risk of haemorrhage, infection, or a history of adverse pregnancy outcomes. Review the woman's condition after 7 to 14 days.
  - **Follow-Up:** If bleeding and pain do not start or continue, or if the miscarriage seems incomplete, discuss all options (expectant, medical, and surgical) with the woman.
- **Medical Management:**
  - **Misoprostol Use:** Offer vaginal misoprostol (800 micrograms) for missed or incomplete miscarriage. Oral misoprostol is an acceptable alternative. For incomplete miscarriages, a single dose of 600 micrograms (or 800 micrograms) is used.
  - **Information:** Inform women about the expected process, including bleeding duration and potential side effects (pain, diarrhoea, vomiting). Provide pain relief and anti-emetics as needed. Advise follow-up if a positive pregnancy test remains after 3 weeks to rule out molar or ectopic pregnancy.

- **Surgical Management:**
  - **Options:** Offer manual vacuum aspiration (MVA) under local anaesthesia in an outpatient setting or surgical management under general anaesthesia. Provide detailed oral and written information about the procedures.
  - **Criteria for Outpatient MVA:** Include being hemodynamically stable, parous, well-motivated, and having an early fetal demise with CRL <25 mm or incomplete miscarriage with retained products <5 cm. Exclude cases with a gestational period >10 weeks, panic attacks, cervical stenosis, large fibroids, or other contraindications.

Single Best Answer (SBA) Questions

SBA 71

A 30-year-old woman presents with a 6-week history of amenorrhoea, pelvic pain, and vaginal bleeding. Her β-hCG level is 1500 IU/L, and a transvaginal ultrasound shows an empty uterus. Which of the following is the most likely diagnosis?

a) Complete miscarriage

b) Ectopic pregnancy

c) Molar pregnancy

d) Threatened miscarriage

e) Normal early pregnancy

SBA 72

A 28-year-old woman presents with severe right lower abdominal pain and vaginal bleeding at 8 weeks of gestation. Her β-hCG is 3000 IU/L, and transvaginal ultrasound reveals a complex adnexal mass with free fluid in the pelvis. What is the most appropriate next step?

a) Expectant management

b) Methotrexate therapy

c) Laparoscopic salpingectomy

d) Repeat ultrasound in one week

e) Oral progesterone therapy

SBA 73

A 32-year-old woman with a history of pelvic inflammatory disease (PID) presents with sudden-onset left-sided pelvic pain at 7 weeks of gestation. Ultrasound confirms a left-sided ectopic pregnancy. What is the most likely reason for her ectopic pregnancy?

a) Smoking

b) Previous tubal surgery

c) Endometriosis

d) History of PID

e) Previous caesarean section

SBA 74

A 29-year-old woman with a confirmed ectopic pregnancy has a β-hCG level of 3500 IU/L and an adnexal mass of 30 mm on ultrasound. She is hemodynamically stable with no signs of rupture. What is the best initial management?

a) Expectant management

b) Methotrexate therapy

c) Laparotomy

d) Salpingectomy

e) Salpingotomy

SBA 75

A 35-year-old woman presents with amenorrhoea, light vaginal bleeding, and pelvic pain. Her ultrasound shows an empty uterine cavity and a 20 mm gestational sac in the cervix. Which of the following best describes her condition?

a) Cervical ectopic pregnancy

b) Molar pregnancy

c) Complete miscarriage

d) Heterotopic pregnancy

e) Cornual ectopic pregnancy

SBA 76

Which of the following is the most accurate method for dating a pregnancy up to 13+6 weeks?

a) Mean sac diameter

b) Crown-rump length (CRL)

c) Head circumference

d) Biparietal diameter

e) Femur length

SBA 77

A 25-year-old woman at 10 weeks of gestation presents with vaginal bleeding and cramping. An ultrasound shows a fetal pole with a CRL of 6 mm but no visible heartbeat. What is the next appropriate step?

    a) Immediate surgical management

    b) Reassure and discharge

    c) Offer medical management with misoprostol

    d) Repeat ultrasound in 7 days

    e) Expectant management

SBA 78

A woman with a history of ectopic pregnancy is undergoing an early pregnancy scan. Which of the following ultrasound findings most strongly suggests an ectopic pregnancy?

    a) Empty uterus with a pseudogestational sac

    b) Yolk sac in the uterus

    c) Free fluid in the pouch of Douglas

    d) Gestational sac with fetal pole in the uterus

    e) Complex adnexal mass separate from the ovary

SBA 79

A 33-year-old woman with a positive pregnancy test and 8 weeks of amenorrhoea presents with vaginal bleeding. Her ultrasound shows an empty uterus. What is the next best step in her management?

a) Start progesterone therapy

b) Advise expectant management

c) Repeat β-hCG in 48 hours

d) Immediate surgical intervention

e) Prescribe misoprostol

SBA 80

A woman with a known intrauterine pregnancy at 9 weeks of gestation presents with light vaginal bleeding. An ultrasound confirms a viable fetus with a heartbeat. What is the most appropriate advice?

a) Immediate surgical intervention

b) Start bed rest and avoid physical activity

c) Expectant management with follow-up if bleeding persists

d) Initiate progesterone supplementation

e) Repeat ultrasound in 48 hours

SBA 81

A 26-year-old woman with a history of a caesarean section presents with lower abdominal pain at 6 weeks of gestation. Her ultrasound shows a gestational sac located in the lower uterine segment. Which of the following best describes her condition?

a) Cervical ectopic pregnancy

b) Normal intrauterine pregnancy

c) Cornual ectopic pregnancy

d) Caesarean section scar ectopic pregnancy

e) Interstitial ectopic pregnancy

SBA 82

A 27-year-old woman at 7 weeks of gestation presents with abdominal pain and vaginal bleeding. Her β-hCG level is 8000 IU/L. An ultrasound shows a gestational sac in the cornual region of the uterus. What is the most appropriate management?

a) Expectant management

b) Methotrexate therapy

c) Laparoscopic cornual resection

d) Manual vacuum aspiration

e) Prescribe oral progesterone

SBA 83

A 24-year-old woman at 10 weeks of gestation presents with sudden severe abdominal pain and dizziness. Her vital signs show hypotension and tachycardia. Ultrasound reveals free fluid in the abdomen and an adnexal mass. What is the next best step?

    a) Methotrexate therapy

    b) Salpingotomy

    c) Immediate laparoscopy

    d) Expectant management

    e) Serial β-hCG monitoring

SBA 84

Which of the following is the most common site of implantation in an ectopic pregnancy?

    a) Cervix

    b) Ampulla of the fallopian tube

    c) Ovary

    d) Interstitial part of the fallopian tube

    e) Fimbriae of the fallopian tube

SBA 85

A 32-year-old woman presents with a positive pregnancy test and a history of previous ectopic pregnancy. Which of the following is the most appropriate method for early confirmation of an intrauterine pregnancy?

a) Serial β-hCG measurements

b) Transabdominal ultrasound at 8 weeks

c) Early transvaginal ultrasound

d) Clinical examination

e) Wait until 12 weeks for the dating scan

SBA 86

A 28-year-old woman with a known ectopic pregnancy has a β-hCG level of 5000 IU/L and an adnexal mass of 40 mm. She is stable with no signs of rupture. What is the best management option?

a) Expectant management

b) Methotrexate therapy

c) Salpingectomy

d) Laparotomy

e) Salpingotomy

SBA 87

A woman with a known intrauterine pregnancy presents with severe lower abdominal pain and dizziness at 8 weeks of gestation. An ultrasound shows a viable intrauterine pregnancy and a large amount of free fluid in the abdomen. What is the most likely diagnosis?

a) Appendicitis

b) Ruptured ovarian cyst

c) Heterotopic pregnancy

d) Ectopic pregnancy

e) Normal pregnancy

SBA 88

A 30-year-old woman presents with amenorrhoea, vaginal bleeding, and a positive pregnancy test. Transvaginal ultrasound shows a thickened endometrium with no gestational sac. What is the most appropriate next step?

a) Repeat ultrasound in 2 weeks

b) Immediate surgical evacuation

c) Serial β-hCG measurements

d) Start progesterone therapy

e) Administer methotrexate

SBA 89

A 27-year-old woman presents at 9 weeks of gestation with spotting. An ultrasound shows a viable intrauterine pregnancy with a heartbeat and a subchorionic hematoma. What is the recommended management?

a) Immediate surgical evacuation

b) Administer progesterone

c) Expectant management

d) Start bed rest

e) Repeat ultrasound in 2 weeks

SBA 90

A 31-year-old woman with a confirmed intrauterine pregnancy at 7 weeks of gestation presents with right-sided pelvic pain and a history of tubal surgery. What is the most appropriate investigation to rule out an ectopic pregnancy?

a) Transabdominal ultrasound

b) MRI pelvis

c) Serum progesterone level

d) Laparoscopy

e) Transvaginal ultrasound

SBA 91

A 26-year-old woman presents with heavy vaginal bleeding and cramping at 10 weeks of gestation. An ultrasound shows an empty uterus with some retained products of conception. What is the most appropriate next step?

a) Administer methotrexate

b) Expectant management

c) Surgical evacuation

d) Repeat β-hCG in 48 hours

e) Start progesterone therapy

SBA 92

A 31-year-old woman with a previous cesarean section presents at 7 weeks gestation with a gestational sac located in the lower uterine segment on ultrasound, suggestive of a cesarean section scar ectopic pregnancy. Her β-hCG level is 4000 IU/L, and she is hemodynamically stable. Which is the most appropriate management option?

a) Expectant management
b) Methotrexate therapy
c) Laparoscopic removal
d) Dilation and curettage
e) Surgical resection

SBA 93

A 28-year-old woman at 7 weeks of gestation presents with heavy vaginal bleeding and severe cramping. Ultrasound reveals a gestational sac with a fetal pole measuring 25 mm without a heartbeat. What is the most appropriate management?

a) Expectant management

b) Misoprostol therapy

c) Surgical evacuation

d) Methotrexate therapy

e) Bed rest and observation

SBA 94

A woman with a confirmed intrauterine pregnancy presents with spotting at 9 weeks. An ultrasound reveals a viable fetus with a small subchorionic hemorrhage. What is the most likely outcome?

a) Complete miscarriage

b) Threatened miscarriage

c) Ectopic pregnancy

d) Molar pregnancy

e) Normal pregnancy

SBA 95

A 30-year-old woman at 6 weeks gestation presents with spotting and mild cramping. A transvaginal ultrasound shows a gestational sac with a CRL of 5 mm but no visible heartbeat. What is the most appropriate follow-up?

a) Immediate surgical management

b) Reassess with ultrasound in 7 days

c) Initiate progesterone therapy

d) Expectant management for miscarriage

e) Serial β-hCG measurements

SBA 96

A 29-year-old woman presents with vaginal bleeding and cramping at 11 weeks gestation. Ultrasound shows a CRL of 15 mm but no heartbeat. What is the most likely diagnosis?

a) Threatened miscarriage

b) Missed miscarriage

c) Complete miscarriage

d) Ectopic pregnancy

e) Molar pregnancy

SBA 97

A 35-year-old woman presents with amenorrhoea and a positive pregnancy test. Her last menstrual period was 12 weeks ago. Ultrasound shows a 25 mm gestational sac with no fetal pole. What is the most appropriate next step?

a) Serial β-hCG monitoring

b) Expectant management

c) Reassess with ultrasound in 7 days

d) Surgical management

e) Initiate methotrexate therapy

SBA 98

Which of the following factors is most likely to influence the choice between medical and surgical management of a missed miscarriage?

a) Gestational age

b) Patient's preference

c) Presence of infection

d) Previous miscarriage history

e) CRL measurement

SBA 99

A 31-year-old woman at 8 weeks gestation presents with vaginal bleeding. An ultrasound shows a viable pregnancy but with a 20 mm subchorionic hemorrhage. What is the appropriate management plan?

a) Immediate surgical evacuation

b) Bed rest and follow-up ultrasound

c) Expectant management

d) Start oral progesterone

e) Initiate misoprostol therapy

SBA 100

A woman presents with spotting and a positive pregnancy test at 5 weeks gestation. Transvaginal ultrasound shows an empty gestational sac with a mean diameter of 18 mm. What is the most appropriate follow-up?

a) Expectant management

b) Reassess with ultrasound in 7 days

c) Immediate surgical evacuation

d) Serial β-hCG monitoring

e) Prescribe progesterone therapy

SBA 101

A 27-year-old woman with a known history of ectopic pregnancy presents with left-sided pelvic pain at 6 weeks gestation. Ultrasound shows an intrauterine gestational sac and a complex adnexal mass. What is the most likely diagnosis?

    a) Ovarian cyst

    b) Heterotopic pregnancy

    c) Normal early pregnancy

    d) Molar pregnancy

    e) Cervical ectopic pregnancy

SBA 102

A 32-year-old woman at 8 weeks gestation presents with vaginal bleeding. Ultrasound shows a CRL of 8 mm without a heartbeat. What is the most appropriate next step?

    a) Offer medical management with misoprostol

    b) Immediate surgical management

    c) Reassess with ultrasound in 7 days

    d) Expectant management

    e) Start oral progesterone

SBA 103

A woman at 7 weeks gestation presents with vaginal bleeding and cramping. Ultrasound shows an intrauterine gestational sac with a CRL of 7 mm but no heartbeat. What is the most likely diagnosis?

a) Complete miscarriage

b) Missed miscarriage

c) Threatened miscarriage

d) Ectopic pregnancy

e) Molar pregnancy

SBA 104

A 33-year-old woman presents at 9 weeks gestation with severe cramping and vaginal bleeding. Ultrasound shows retained products of conception in the uterus. What is the most appropriate next step?

a) Administer methotrexate

b) Expectant management

c) Surgical evacuation

d) Repeat β-hCG in 48 hours

e) Start oral progesterone

SBA 105

A 26-year-old woman presents with lower abdominal pain and vaginal bleeding at 8 weeks gestation. Ultrasound shows a viable intrauterine pregnancy and a small amount of free fluid in the pouch of Douglas. What is the most likely diagnosis?

a) Threatened miscarriage

b) Ectopic pregnancy

c) Heterotopic pregnancy

d) Ovarian torsion

e) Normal pregnancy

SBA 106

A woman presents with vaginal bleeding and cramping at 10 weeks gestation. Ultrasound shows a gestational sac with a fetal pole measuring 20 mm and no heartbeat. What is the most appropriate management?

a) Expectant management

b) Misoprostol therapy

c) Surgical evacuation

d) Bed rest and follow-up

e) Serial β-hCG monitoring

SBA 107

A 35-year-old woman with a history of recurrent miscarriages presents with spotting at 6 weeks gestation. An ultrasound shows a gestational sac and yolk sac but no fetal pole. What is the most appropriate follow-up?

a) Expectant management

b) Reassess with ultrasound in 7 days

c) Immediate surgical evacuation

d) Serial β-hCG monitoring

e) Start progesterone therapy

SBA 108

A 29-year-old woman at 11 weeks gestation presents with heavy vaginal bleeding and severe cramping. Ultrasound shows a retained gestational sac with no heartbeat. What is the most appropriate management?

a) Administer methotrexate

b) Expectant management

c) Misoprostol therapy

d) Surgical evacuation

e) Bed rest and observation

SBA 109

A 32-year-old woman with a known intrauterine pregnancy presents with sudden lower abdominal pain and vaginal bleeding at 8 weeks gestation. Ultrasound reveals an intrauterine gestational sac and a small amount of free fluid in the abdomen. What is the most likely diagnosis?

    a) Threatened miscarriage

    b) Ectopic pregnancy

    c) Heterotopic pregnancy

    d) Appendicitis

    e) Normal pregnancy

SBA 110

A 27-year-old woman presents with severe lower abdominal pain at 7 weeks gestation. Ultrasound shows an empty uterus with a complex adnexal mass. What is the most likely diagnosis?

    a) Molar pregnancy

    b) Ectopic pregnancy

    c) Threatened miscarriage

    d) Complete miscarriage

    e) Normal early pregnancy

SBA 111

A woman at 8 weeks gestation presents with spotting. An ultrasound reveals a CRL of 8 mm but no visible heartbeat. What is the most appropriate next step?

a) Immediate surgical management

b) Reassess with ultrasound in 7 days

c) Administer methotrexate

d) Expectant management

e) Start oral progesterone

SBA 112

A 30-year-old woman presents with vaginal bleeding at 12 weeks gestation. Ultrasound shows a gestational sac with no fetal pole and a mean sac diameter of 35 mm. What is the most appropriate diagnosis?

a) Threatened miscarriage

b) Missed miscarriage

c) Complete miscarriage

d) Ectopic pregnancy

e) Normal pregnancy

SBA 113

A 31-year-old woman at 9 weeks gestation presents with heavy vaginal bleeding. Ultrasound shows an empty uterus with some retained products of conception. What is the most appropriate management?

a) Expectant management

b) Misoprostol therapy

c) Surgical evacuation

d) Administer methotrexate

e) Start oral progesterone

SBA 114

A 28-year-old woman presents with severe pelvic pain at 7 weeks gestation. Ultrasound shows an empty uterus and a right adnexal mass. What is the most likely diagnosis?

a) Complete miscarriage

b) Ectopic pregnancy

c) Threatened miscarriage

d) Molar pregnancy

e) Normal early pregnancy

SBA 115

Which of the following is the most common site of ectopic pregnancy implantation?

A) Cervix

B) Ovary

C) Ampullary section of the fallopian tube

D) Interstitial part of the tube

E) Abdominal cavity

SBA 116

In the UK, what is the approximate incidence of ectopic pregnancy among pregnancies?

A) 1 in 100

B) 11 in 1000

C) 1 in 500

D) 5 in 1000

E) 15 in 100

SBA 117

A 34-year-old woman with a confirmed ectopic pregnancy presents with a stable hemodynamic status. Her serum β-hCG level is 1500 IU/L, and the ectopic mass is 2 cm in size. What is the most appropriate management?

A) Laparotomy

B) Expectant management

C) Methotrexate administration

D) Salpingectomy

E) Referral for IVF

SBA 118

What percentage of ectopic pregnancies occurs without any known risk factors?

A) 10%

B) 25%

C) 33%

D) 50%

E) 75%

SBA 119

Which of the following is the most significant risk factor for the recurrence of an ectopic pregnancy?

A) Smoking

B) Previous ectopic pregnancy

C) Use of intrauterine devices (IUDs)

D) Tubal surgery

E) Pelvic inflammatory disease (PID)

SBA 120

A 30-year-old woman presents with amenorrhoea and lower abdominal pain. A transvaginal ultrasound reveals an empty uterus. What is the next best step in managing this patient?

A) Perform a serum β-hCG test

B) Reassure and discharge

C) Schedule a follow-up ultrasound in 14 days

D) Immediate laparoscopic exploration

E) Prescribe methotrexate

Extended Match Questions (EMQ)

EMQ 21

Question: Identify the most appropriate management or diagnostic action based on the clinical scenario:

1. A 30-year-old at 8 weeks gestation presents with a CRL of 7 mm but no visible heartbeat on transvaginal ultrasound.
2. A 28-year-old at 10 weeks gestation presents with vaginal bleeding, and the ultrasound shows an empty gestational sac measuring 26 mm.
3. A 32-year-old at 7 weeks gestation presents with a sac diameter of 24 mm without a fetal pole.
4. A 26-year-old at 9 weeks gestation with a confirmed intrauterine pregnancy and fetal heartbeat complains of mild spotting.
5. A 33-year-old at 12 weeks gestation presents with abdominal pain. The ultrasound shows a complex adnexal mass with no intrauterine pregnancy.

Options:

A) Expectant management
B) Surgical management
C) Medical management with misoprostol
D) Repeat ultrasound in 7 days
E) Reassurance and routine antenatal care
F) Laparoscopy
G) Serial β-hCG measurement
H) Immediate referral to early pregnancy assessment service

EMQ 22

Question: Choose the most appropriate intervention or diagnostic test for the following scenarios:

1. A 35-year-old woman with a history of recurrent miscarriages presents at 8 weeks with vaginal bleeding. Ultrasound shows a gestational sac of 22 mm without a fetal pole.
2. A 29-year-old at 6 weeks gestation presents with spotting. Ultrasound shows a gestational sac with a yolk sac but no fetal pole.
3. A 27-year-old at 7 weeks gestation presents with mild cramping. Ultrasound shows a CRL of 6 mm without visible cardiac activity.
4. A 31-year-old at 10 weeks gestation with a previous history of molar pregnancy presents with heavy bleeding. Ultrasound shows an empty uterus.
5. A 28-year-old at 9 weeks gestation presents with mild bleeding. Ultrasound shows a fetal heartbeat and subchorionic hemorrhage.

Options:

A) Expectant management
B) Surgical evacuation
C) Reassurance and routine antenatal care
D) Laparoscopy
E) Repeat ultrasound in 7 days
F) Serial β-hCG measurement
G) Immediate referral to early pregnancy assessment service

EMQ 23

Question: Match the clinical presentation with the most appropriate diagnostic action or management:

1. A 32-year-old at 7 weeks gestation with a gestational sac diameter of 25 mm but no fetal pole.
2. A 29-year-old at 9 weeks gestation with a CRL of 7 mm and no visible fetal heartbeat.
3. A 26-year-old at 6 weeks gestation presents with severe abdominal pain and spotting. Ultrasound shows a complex adnexal mass.
4. A 34-year-old at 11 weeks gestation presents with spotting and a gestational sac of 20 mm without a fetal pole.
5. A 30-year-old at 8 weeks gestation presents with light vaginal bleeding and a confirmed intrauterine pregnancy with a heartbeat.

Options:

A) Repeat ultrasound in 7 days
B) Expectant management
C) Surgical evacuation
D) Laparoscopy
E) Serial β-hCG measurement
F) Reassurance and routine antenatal care
G) Immediate referral to early pregnancy assessment service

EMQ 24

Question: Identify the most appropriate diagnostic follow-up or management for each scenario:

1. A 29-year-old at 8 weeks gestation with a confirmed intrauterine pregnancy and mild bleeding.
2. A 31-year-old at 9 weeks gestation with no visible fetal pole but a sac diameter of 27 mm.
3. A 33-year-old at 10 weeks gestation with a CRL of 8 mm without visible fetal heart activity.

4. A 27-year-old at 7 weeks gestation with severe abdominal pain and an ultrasound showing a complex adnexal mass.
5. A 32-year-old at 8 weeks gestation with a yolk sac but no fetal pole on ultrasound.

Options:

A) Serial β-hCG measurement
B) Repeat ultrasound in 7 days
C) Surgical evacuation
D) Laparoscopy
E) Expectant management
F) Immediate referral to early pregnancy assessment service
G) Reassurance and routine antenatal care

EMQ 25

Question: Choose the most appropriate next step for each clinical scenario:

1. A 28-year-old at 6 weeks gestation presents with mild spotting. Ultrasound shows a CRL of 5 mm but no visible heartbeat.
2. A 30-year-old at 9 weeks gestation presents with an empty gestational sac of 30 mm without a fetal pole.
3. A 32-year-old at 7 weeks gestation presents with abdominal pain. Ultrasound shows an empty uterus and complex adnexal mass.
4. A 31-year-old at 10 weeks gestation presents with heavy bleeding. Ultrasound shows an empty gestational sac of 27 mm.
5. A 29-year-old at 8 weeks gestation presents with a confirmed intrauterine pregnancy and fetal heartbeat, but reports mild bleeding.

Options:

A) Expectant management
B) Surgical management
C) Medical management with misoprostol
D) Repeat ultrasound in 7 days
E) Reassurance and routine antenatal care
F) Laparoscopy
G) Serial β-hCG measurement

EMQ 26

Question: Identify the most appropriate next step in management or diagnosis based on the clinical scenario:

1. A 34-year-old at 8 weeks gestation presents with heavy vaginal bleeding and a CRL of 8 mm without visible heartbeat.
2. A 28-year-old at 9 weeks gestation presents with mild cramping and an ultrasound showing a gestational sac of 24 mm with no fetal pole.
3. A 30-year-old at 6 weeks gestation presents with spotting. Ultrasound shows an empty gestational sac of 26 mm.
4. A 35-year-old at 10 weeks gestation presents with severe abdominal pain and a complex adnexal mass on ultrasound.
5. A 29-year-old at 7 weeks gestation presents with mild bleeding and an ultrasound showing a confirmed fetal heartbeat.

Options:

A) Serial β-hCG measurement
B) Repeat ultrasound in 7 days
C) Expectant management
D) Laparoscopy

E) Surgical management
F) Medical management with misoprostol
G) Reassurance and routine antenatal care

EMQ 27

Question: Choose the most appropriate management or diagnostic approach for the following scenarios:

1. A 26-year-old at 7 weeks gestation with a history of recurrent miscarriages presents with mild spotting. Ultrasound shows a fetal pole of 6 mm with no visible heartbeat.
2. A 30-year-old at 10 weeks gestation presents with an empty gestational sac of 28 mm without a fetal pole.
3. A 32-year-old at 8 weeks gestation presents with severe abdominal pain. Ultrasound shows a complex adnexal mass with no intrauterine pregnancy.
4. A 29-year-old at 9 weeks gestation presents with mild bleeding and an ultrasound showing a confirmed fetal heartbeat.
5. A 31-year-old at 11 weeks gestation presents with heavy bleeding. Ultrasound shows an empty gestational sac of 26 mm.

Options:

A) Repeat ultrasound in 7 days
B) Laparoscopy
C) Serial β-hCG measurement
D) Surgical management
E) Reassurance and routine antenatal care
F) Expectant management
G) Immediate referral to early pregnancy assessment service

EMQ 28

Question: Match the clinical scenario with the most appropriate management plan:

1. A 32-year-old at 8 weeks gestation presents with a CRL of 6 mm without a visible heartbeat.
2. A 28-year-old at 9 weeks gestation presents with heavy bleeding and an ultrasound showing a gestational sac of 25 mm with no fetal pole.
3. A 30-year-old at 7 weeks gestation with a history of ectopic pregnancy presents with severe lower abdominal pain. Ultrasound shows a complex adnexal mass.
4. A 26-year-old at 6 weeks gestation presents with mild cramping and an ultrasound showing a confirmed fetal heartbeat.
5. A 31-year-old at 10 weeks gestation presents with spotting. Ultrasound shows a gestational sac of 28 mm with a yolk sac but no fetal pole.

Options:

A) Surgical management
B) Laparoscopy
C) Serial β-hCG measurement
D) Expectant management
E) Reassurance and routine antenatal care
F) Repeat ultrasound in 7 days
G) Immediate referral to early pregnancy assessment service

EMQ 29

Question: Determine the most appropriate next step based on the clinical scenario:

1. A 35-year-old at 9 weeks gestation presents with a CRL of 9 mm with no visible fetal heartbeat on ultrasound.
2. A 30-year-old at 6 weeks gestation presents with spotting and a confirmed fetal heartbeat on ultrasound.
3. A 33-year-old at 7 weeks gestation presents with severe lower abdominal pain. Ultrasound shows a complex adnexal mass.
4. A 27-year-old at 8 weeks gestation presents with mild bleeding and an ultrasound showing a yolk sac but no fetal pole.
5. A 28-year-old at 10 weeks gestation presents with an empty gestational sac of 26 mm without a fetal pole.

Options:

A) Serial β-hCG measurement
B) Repeat ultrasound in 7 days
C) Expectant management
D) Surgical management
E) Laparoscopy
F) Reassurance and routine antenatal care
G) Medical management with misoprostol

EMQ 30

Question: Match the clinical presentation with the most appropriate diagnostic or management approach:

1. A 29-year-old at 8 weeks gestation presents with spotting. Ultrasound shows a CRL of 6 mm but no visible heartbeat.

2. A 31-year-old at 9 weeks gestation presents with heavy bleeding. Ultrasound shows an empty gestational sac of 30 mm without a fetal pole.
3. A 26-year-old at 7 weeks gestation presents with severe abdominal pain and an ultrasound showing a complex adnexal mass.
4. A 30-year-old at 10 weeks gestation presents with a gestational sac of 28 mm with a yolk sac but no fetal pole.
5. A 27-year-old at 6 weeks gestation presents with mild spotting and an ultrasound showing a confirmed fetal heartbeat.

Options:

A) Laparoscopy
B) Surgical management
C) Medical management with misoprostol
D) Repeat ultrasound in 7 days
E) Reassurance and routine antenatal care
F) Serial β-hCG measurement
G) Expectant management

EMQ 31

Question: Determine the most appropriate next step in management or diagnosis for each scenario:

1. A 27-year-old woman at 8 weeks gestation presents with vaginal bleeding. Ultrasound shows a CRL of 5 mm without a visible heartbeat.

2. A 32-year-old woman at 9 weeks gestation presents with mild abdominal pain and an ultrasound showing a gestational sac of 23 mm with no fetal pole.

3. A 30-year-old woman at 10 weeks gestation presents with severe abdominal pain and ultrasound findings of a complex adnexal mass.

4. A 29-year-old woman at 7 weeks gestation presents with mild bleeding and an ultrasound showing a confirmed fetal heartbeat.

5. A 35-year-old woman at 6 weeks gestation presents with heavy bleeding. Ultrasound shows an empty uterus.

Options:

A) Repeat ultrasound in 7 days
B) Surgical management
C) Expectant management
D) Laparoscopy
E) Serial β-hCG measurement
F) Reassurance and routine antenatal care

EMQ 32

Question: Identify the most appropriate diagnostic or follow-up action for each scenario:

1. A 34-year-old woman at 9 weeks gestation presents with vaginal bleeding and a CRL of 7 mm with no visible heartbeat on transvaginal ultrasound.

2. A 28-year-old woman at 8 weeks gestation presents with an ultrasound showing a gestational sac of 26 mm with no fetal pole.

3. A 31-year-old woman at 7 weeks gestation presents with no symptoms, and ultrasound reveals a gestational sac but no yolk sac or fetal pole.

4. A 29-year-old woman at 11 weeks gestation presents with spotting. Ultrasound shows a gestational sac with a fetal pole but no heartbeat.

5. A 26-year-old woman at 6 weeks gestation presents with lower abdominal pain and ultrasound shows a gestational sac without a fetal pole. β-hCG is 3000 IU/L.

Options:

A) Repeat scan in 7 days
B) Laparoscopy
C) Serial β-hCG measurement
D) Surgical management
E) Reassurance and routine antenatal care
F) Expectant management
G) Immediate referral to early pregnancy assessment service

EMQ 33

Question: Match the clinical presentation with the most appropriate management plan:

1. A 30-year-old woman at 8 weeks gestation presents with spotting. Ultrasound shows a CRL of 7 mm without a visible heartbeat.

2. A 32-year-old woman at 9 weeks gestation presents with heavy bleeding. Ultrasound shows an empty gestational sac of 29 mm without a fetal pole.

3. A 28-year-old woman at 7 weeks gestation with a history of ectopic pregnancy presents with severe lower abdominal pain. Ultrasound shows a complex adnexal mass.

4. A 26-year-old woman at 6 weeks gestation presents with mild cramping and an ultrasound showing a confirmed fetal heartbeat.

5. A 31-year-old woman at 10 weeks gestation presents with spotting. Ultrasound shows a gestational sac of 27 mm with a yolk sac but no fetal pole.

Options:

A) Surgical management
B) Laparoscopy
C) Serial β-hCG measurement
D) Expectant management
E) Reassurance and routine antenatal care
F) Repeat ultrasound in 7 days
G) Medical management with misoprostol

EMQ 34

Question: Select the most appropriate management approach for each scenario:

1. A 29-year-old woman at 7 weeks gestation presents with mild bleeding. Ultrasound shows a gestational sac with a yolk sac but no fetal pole.

2. A 31-year-old woman at 10 weeks gestation presents with an empty gestational sac of 26 mm without a fetal pole.

3. A 35-year-old woman at 8 weeks gestation presents with a CRL of 9 mm without a visible heartbeat on ultrasound.

4. A 32-year-old woman at 6 weeks gestation presents with lower abdominal pain. Ultrasound shows an empty uterus with an adnexal mass.

5. A 30-year-old woman at 9 weeks gestation presents with spotting. Ultrasound shows a confirmed fetal heartbeat.

Options:

A) Laparoscopy
B) Surgical management
C) Medical management with misoprostol
D) Repeat ultrasound in 7 days
E) Reassurance and routine antenatal care
F) Serial β-hCG measurement
G) Expectant management

EMQ 35

Question: Match the clinical scenario with the most appropriate management or diagnostic approach:

1. A 34-year-old woman at 10 weeks gestation presents with a gestational sac of 28 mm with no fetal pole or yolk sac.

2. A 29-year-old woman at 8 weeks gestation presents with spotting. Ultrasound shows a CRL of 7 mm with no visible heartbeat.

3. A 28-year-old woman at 9 weeks gestation presents with heavy bleeding and an ultrasound showing an empty gestational sac of 30 mm without a fetal pole.

4. A 30-year-old woman at 6 weeks gestation presents with lower abdominal pain and an ultrasound showing an empty uterus with a β-hCG of 2000 IU/L.

5. A 31-year-old woman at 7 weeks gestation presents with mild cramping and an ultrasound showing a confirmed fetal heartbeat.

Options:

A) Laparoscopy
B) Serial β-hCG measurement
C) Repeat ultrasound in 7 days
D) Surgical management
E) Expectant management
F) Medical management with misoprostol
G) Reassurance and routine antenatal care

EMQ 36

Question: Match each clinical scenario with the most appropriate management plan:

1. A 29-year-old woman at 8 weeks gestation presents with vaginal bleeding. Ultrasound shows a CRL of 8 mm with no visible heartbeat.

2. A 30-year-old woman at 9 weeks gestation presents with an ultrasound showing a gestational sac of 27 mm without a fetal pole.

3. A 31-year-old woman at 7 weeks gestation presents with mild abdominal pain and an ultrasound showing a complex adnexal mass.

4. A 28-year-old woman at 6 weeks gestation presents with an ultrasound showing an empty gestational sac and β-hCG of 2500 IU/L.

5. A 35-year-old woman at 10 weeks gestation presents with severe bleeding. Ultrasound shows an empty uterus.

Options:

A) Serial β-hCG measurement
B) Surgical management
C) Expectant management

D) Laparoscopy
E) Repeat ultrasound in 7 days
F) Reassurance and routine antenatal care

EMQ 37

Question: Determine the most appropriate diagnostic or follow-up action for each scenario:

1. A 33-year-old woman at 7 weeks gestation presents with a CRL of 6 mm and no visible heartbeat on transvaginal ultrasound.

2. A 28-year-old woman at 8 weeks gestation presents with an ultrasound showing a gestational sac of 22 mm with no fetal pole.

3. A 31-year-old woman at 9 weeks gestation presents with spotting and an ultrasound showing a fetal pole but no heartbeat.

4. A 30-year-old woman at 10 weeks gestation presents with lower abdominal pain and an ultrasound showing a gestational sac without a fetal pole.

5. A 27-year-old woman at 6 weeks gestation presents with an ultrasound showing an empty gestational sac and β-hCG of 1500 IU/L.

Options:

A) Serial β-hCG measurement
B) Laparoscopy
C) Surgical management
D) Repeat ultrasound in 7 days
E) Reassurance and routine antenatal care
F) Expectant management

EMQ 38

Question: Match the clinical scenario with the most appropriate treatment option:

1. A 30-year-old woman at 7 weeks gestation presents with vaginal bleeding and an ultrasound showing a CRL of 7 mm with no visible heartbeat.

2. A 32-year-old woman at 9 weeks gestation presents with severe bleeding and an ultrasound showing an empty gestational sac of 30 mm without a fetal pole.

3. A 28-year-old woman at 8 weeks gestation presents with severe lower abdominal pain and an ultrasound showing a complex adnexal mass.

4. A 26-year-old woman at 6 weeks gestation presents with an ultrasound showing a confirmed fetal heartbeat and mild cramping.

5. A 29-year-old woman at 8 weeks gestation presents with spotting. Ultrasound shows a gestational sac of 28 mm with no fetal pole.

Options:

A) Surgical management
B) Laparoscopy
C) Medical management with misoprostol
D) Expectant management
E) Reassurance and routine antenatal care
F) Repeat ultrasound in 7 days
G) Serial β-hCG measurement

EMQ 39

Question: Select the most appropriate management strategy for each scenario:

1. A 31-year-old woman at 10 weeks gestation presents with spotting and an ultrasound showing a CRL of 9 mm with no visible heartbeat.

2. A 30-year-old woman at 8 weeks gestation presents with an ultrasound showing a gestational sac of 25 mm with no fetal pole.

3. A 35-year-old woman at 7 weeks gestation presents with severe bleeding and an ultrasound showing an empty uterus.

4. A 28-year-old woman at 6 weeks gestation presents with an ultrasound showing an empty gestational sac and β-hCG of 2000 IU/L.

5. A 29-year-old woman at 9 weeks gestation presents with spotting and an ultrasound showing a confirmed fetal heartbeat.

Options:

A) Laparoscopy
B) Serial β-hCG measurement
C) Surgical management
D) Expectant management
E) Reassurance and routine antenatal care
F) Repeat ultrasound in 7 days

EMQ 40

Question: Determine the appropriate diagnostic or follow-up action for each scenario:

1. A 34-year-old woman at 8 weeks gestation presents with vaginal bleeding. Ultrasound shows a gestational sac of 26 mm without a fetal pole.

2. A 29-year-old woman at 7 weeks gestation presents with spotting and an ultrasound showing a CRL of 6 mm without a visible heartbeat.

3. A 30-year-old woman at 10 weeks gestation presents with heavy bleeding. Ultrasound shows a gestational sac of 28 mm with a yolk sac but no fetal pole.

4. A 27-year-old woman at 6 weeks gestation presents with an ultrasound showing an empty uterus and a β-hCG of 1500 IU/L.

5. A 31-year-old woman at 9 weeks gestation presents with mild cramping and an ultrasound showing a confirmed fetal heartbeat.

Options:

A) Laparoscopy
B) Surgical management
C) Serial β-hCG measurement
D) Expectant management
E) Repeat ultrasound in 7 days
F) Reassurance and routine antenatal care

Anti-D Prophylaxis

1. Timing and Administration:

- **Administration Window:** Anti-D immunoglobulin (Ig) should be administered as soon as possible after potentially sensitising events, and always within 72 hours. If this deadline is missed, protection may still be offered if administered up to 10 days after the event.

2. Potentially Sensitising Events:

- **Procedures and Interventions:**
    - Amniocentesis, chorionic villus sampling, cordocentesis
    - Intrauterine procedures (e.g., therapeutic interventions, surgery)
- **Bleeding and Trauma:**
    - Antepartum haemorrhage, uterine bleeding, abdominal trauma (sharp or blunt)
- **Pregnancy Complications:**
    - Ectopic pregnancy, molar pregnancy evacuation, intrauterine death, stillbirth
- **Delivery:**
    - Normal delivery, instrumental delivery, Caesarean section
- **Other:**
    - External cephalic version, miscarriage, threatened miscarriage.

3. Specific Guidelines for Rh D-Negative Women:

- **General Recommendations:** All non-sensitised Rh D-negative women should receive 250 IU of anti-D Ig.
- **Ectopic Pregnancy:** Anti-D Ig is indicated for surgical management or heavy bleeding. The risk of alloimmunisation from medical or expectant management is low and does not require routine anti-D prophylaxis.
- **Miscarriage and Threatened Miscarriage:**
    - **Below 12 Weeks:** Anti-D Ig is generally not required for a threatened miscarriage or complete miscarriage if below 12 weeks of gestation.
    - **Above 12 Weeks:** Administer 250 IU of anti-D Ig for miscarriages above 12 weeks, and if the miscarriage involves heavy bleeding or severe pain.
- **Intraoperative Cell Salvage:** Anti-D Ig is also recommended if intraoperative cell salvage is used during delivery.

4. Dosage Adjustments:

- **Routine Prophylaxis:** 250 IU of anti-D Ig is administered.
- **Quantifying Fetal-Maternal Haemorrhage:** At 20 weeks or later, or in cases of significant haemorrhage, anti-D Ig dosage may be increased to 500 IU plus a Kleihauer-Betke test to quantify fetal-maternal haemorrhage (FMH).

Single Best Answer (SBA) Questions

SBA 121:
A 28-year-old Rh D-negative woman at 12 weeks gestation presents with mild vaginal bleeding. No fetal heart activity is detected on ultrasound. What is the most appropriate management?
a) Anti-D 250 IU
b) Anti-D 500 IU
c) No anti-D required
d) Anti-D 1500 IU
e) Routine antenatal follow-up

SBA 122:
A 14-week pregnant woman with Rh D-negative blood group undergoes an amniocentesis. What dose of anti-D immunoglobulin should she receive?
a) 100 IU
b) 150 IU
c) 250 IU
d) 500 IU
e) 1500 IU

SBA 123:
A 9-week pregnant Rh D-negative woman experiences a complete miscarriage confirmed by ultrasound. What is the recommended anti-D prophylaxis?
a) Anti-D 250 IU
b) Anti-D 500 IU
c) No anti-D required
d) Anti-D 1500 IU
e) Repeat ultrasound in 7 days

SBA 124:
A 10-week pregnant Rh D-negative woman undergoes a chorionic villus sampling (CVS). What is the appropriate anti-D prophylaxis?
a) Anti-D 100 IU
b) Anti-D 150 IU
c) Anti-D 250 IU
d) Anti-D 500 IU
e) No anti-D required

SBA 125:
A Rh D-negative woman at 20 weeks gestation experiences an abdominal trauma. What is the next best step?
a) Administer 250 IU anti-D
b) Administer 500 IU anti-D
c) Administer 1500 IU anti-D
d) Perform a Kleihauer-Betke test
e) No anti-D required

SBA 126:
A 32-year-old Rh D-negative woman at 28 weeks gestation presents with a threatened miscarriage. What is the most appropriate dose of anti-D prophylaxis?
a) 150 IU
b) 250 IU
c) 500 IU
d) 1500 IU
e) No anti-D required

SBA 127:
A Rh D-negative woman at 22 weeks gestation presents with antepartum haemorrhage. What is the recommended management?

a) Administer 250 IU anti-D
b) Administer 500 IU anti-D
c) Administer 1500 IU anti-D
d) Perform a Kleihauer-Betke test
e) No anti-D required

SBA 128:
A Rh D-negative woman undergoes an external cephalic version at 36 weeks gestation. What is the appropriate anti-D dose?
a) 100 IU
b) 250 IU
c) 500 IU
d) 1500 IU
e) No anti-D required

SBA 129:
A Rh D-negative woman at 15 weeks gestation experiences a significant antepartum haemorrhage. Which test should be performed to quantify fetal-maternal haemorrhage?
a) Kleihauer-Betke test
b) Coombs test
c) ABO typing
d) Rh antibody screen
e) Flow cytometry

SBA 130:
A Rh D-negative woman undergoes an elective Caesarean section at 39 weeks gestation. What is the appropriate anti-D prophylaxis?
a) 250 IU
b) 500 IU
c) 1500 IU

d) 2500 IU
e) No anti-D required

SBA 131:
A 24-year-old Rh D-negative woman presents with abdominal pain at 10 weeks gestation and is diagnosed with an ectopic pregnancy. She undergoes surgical management. What is the appropriate anti-D dose?
a) 150 IU
b) 250 IU
c) 500 IU
d) 1000 IU
e) No anti-D required

SBA 132:
A 34-year-old Rh D-negative woman at 18 weeks gestation undergoes a therapeutic abortion due to severe fetal anomalies. What is the recommended anti-D prophylaxis?
a) 250 IU
b) 500 IU
c) 1000 IU
d) 1500 IU
e) No anti-D required

SBA 133:
A Rh D-negative woman at 24 weeks gestation presents with abdominal trauma after a car accident. What is the appropriate management?
a) Administer 250 IU anti-D
b) Administer 500 IU anti-D
c) Administer 1500 IU anti-D
d) Perform a Kleihauer-Betke test
e) No anti-D required

SBA 134:
A Rh D-negative woman presents with antepartum haemorrhage at 32 weeks gestation. What is the next step in management?
a) Administer 250 IU anti-D
b) Administer 500 IU anti-D
c) Administer 1500 IU anti-D
d) Perform a Kleihauer-Betke test
e) No anti-D required

SBA 135:
A 19-year-old Rh D-negative woman at 8 weeks gestation presents with vaginal bleeding and is diagnosed with a threatened miscarriage. What is the appropriate anti-D management?
a) Anti-D 150 IU
b) Anti-D 250 IU
c) Anti-D 500 IU
d) Anti-D 1000 IU
e) No anti-D required

SBA 136:
A Rh D-negative woman at 22 weeks gestation has an ultrasound showing fetal demise. What is the appropriate management?
a) Administer 250 IU anti-D
b) Administer 500 IU anti-D
c) Administer 1500 IU anti-D
d) Perform a Kleihauer-Betke test
e) No anti-D required

SBA 137:
A 28-year-old Rh D-negative woman presents with vaginal bleeding at 16 weeks gestation. Ultrasound shows an intrauterine pregnancy with fetal heart activity. What is the appropriate anti-D prophylaxis?
a) 250 IU
b) 500 IU
c) 1500 IU
d) 2500 IU
e) No anti-D required

SBA 138:
A Rh D-negative woman at 30 weeks gestation undergoes an amniocentesis. What is the appropriate anti-D prophylaxis?
a) 100 IU
b) 250 IU
c) 500 IU
d) 1000 IU
e) No anti-D required

SBA 139:
A Rh D-negative woman at 36 weeks gestation presents for an elective Caesarean section. What is the appropriate anti-D dose?
a) 250 IU
b) 500 IU
c) 1500 IU
d) 2500 IU
e) No anti-D required

SBA 140:
A Rh D-negative woman at 26 weeks gestation experiences blunt abdominal trauma in a car accident.

What is the most appropriate management?
a) Administer 250 IU anti-D
b) Administer 500 IU anti-D
c) Administer 1500 IU anti-D
d) Perform a Kleihauer-Betke test
e) No anti-D required

Extended Match Questions (EMQ)

EMQ41: Timing and Administration of Anti-D Prophylaxis

Options:

a) Within 72 hours
b) Within 10 days
c) No anti-D required
d) Immediately
e) Within 48 hours

Questions:

1. A 28-year-old Rh D-negative woman presents 9 days after an amniocentesis. What is the appropriate timing for Anti-D prophylaxis?
2. A 32-year-old Rh D-negative woman has a miscarriage at 14 weeks gestation and receives Anti-D 48 hours later. Is this timing appropriate?
3. A 24-year-old woman with a missed miscarriage at 10 weeks gestation and no bleeding is seen. When should Anti-D be administered?
4. A Rh D-negative woman undergoes an external cephalic version at 37 weeks. When should Anti-D be administered?
5. A 26-year-old Rh D-negative woman experiences mild spotting at 6 weeks gestation. Is Anti-D required?

EMQ42: Dosage of Anti-D Prophylaxis

Options:

a) 250 IU

b) 500 IU

c) 1500 IU

d) No Anti-D required

e) 1000 IU

Questions:

1. A Rh D-negative woman undergoes a routine cesarean section at 39 weeks gestation. What dosage of Anti-D is recommended?
2. A 10-week pregnant woman with Rh D-negative blood experiences a miscarriage with moderate bleeding. What dosage of Anti-D is appropriate?
3. After an abdominal trauma at 30 weeks gestation, a Rh D-negative woman undergoes a Kleihauer-Betke test showing significant fetal-maternal haemorrhage. What initial dosage of Anti-D should be given?
4. A Rh D-negative woman has a spontaneous miscarriage at 8 weeks gestation without any bleeding. What is the correct dosage of Anti-D?
5. A Rh D-negative woman undergoes an elective termination of pregnancy at 14 weeks. What dosage of Anti-D should she receive?

EMQ43: Indications for Anti-D Prophylaxis

Options:

a) Ectopic pregnancy managed surgically

b) Threatened miscarriage under 12 weeks with no heavy bleeding

c) Amniocentesis

d) Normal vaginal delivery at term

e) Missed miscarriage at 15 weeks

Questions:

1. A Rh D-negative woman undergoes surgical management for an ectopic pregnancy. Is Anti-D prophylaxis required?
2. A 9-week pregnant Rh D-negative woman with mild spotting has a viable intrauterine pregnancy confirmed by ultrasound. Is Anti-D needed?
3. A Rh D-negative woman has a missed miscarriage at 15 weeks gestation. Is Anti-D required?
4. A Rh D-negative woman undergoes a normal vaginal delivery at 40 weeks. Should Anti-D be administered?
5. A Rh D-negative woman undergoes amniocentesis at 18 weeks gestation. Is Anti-D indicated?

EMQ44: Management of Delayed Anti-D Administration

Options:

a) Administer within 10 days

b) Repeat dose after 24 hours

c) Monitor antibody levels only

d) No further action required

e) Give higher dose of 1500 IU

Questions:

1. A Rh D-negative woman receives Anti-D 7 days after a potentially sensitising event. What should be done next?
2. A Rh D-negative woman who underwent a traumatic delivery receives Anti-D after 8 days. What should be done now?
3. A woman is given a lower dose of Anti-D than required for her gestational age. How should this be managed?
4. Anti-D was administered 11 days after an external cephalic version in a Rh D-negative woman. What is the appropriate management?
5. A Rh D-negative woman who experienced a minor trauma at 30 weeks gestation receives Anti-D within 72 hours. What further action is needed?

EMQ45: Potentially Sensitising Events Requiring Anti-D Prophylaxis

Options:

a) First trimester miscarriage with no bleeding

b) Antepartum haemorrhage after 20 weeks gestation

c) External cephalic version

d) Spontaneous rupture of membranes at term

e) Therapeutic abortion at 8 weeks

Questions:

1. A Rh D-negative woman undergoes an external cephalic version at 36 weeks. Does this event require Anti-D prophylaxis?
2. A 20-week pregnant Rh D-negative woman experiences antepartum haemorrhage. Is Anti-D indicated?
3. A Rh D-negative woman has a spontaneous rupture of membranes at term. Should Anti-D be given?
4. A Rh D-negative woman experiences a first-trimester miscarriage at 7 weeks without any bleeding. Is Anti-D needed?
5. A Rh D-negative woman undergoes a therapeutic abortion at 8 weeks gestation. Should she receive Anti-D?

EMQ46: Indications for Anti-D Prophylaxis

Options:

a) Therapeutic abortion at 9 weeks

b) Spontaneous miscarriage at 6 weeks without bleeding

c) Amniocentesis at 16 weeks

d) Ectopic pregnancy managed with methotrexate

e) External cephalic version at 38 weeks

Questions:

1. A Rh D-negative woman undergoes therapeutic abortion at 9 weeks. Should Anti-D be administered?
2. A Rh D-negative woman has a spontaneous miscarriage at 6 weeks with no bleeding. Is Anti-D required?

3. A Rh D-negative woman undergoes an external cephalic version at 38 weeks. Should she receive Anti-D?
4. A Rh D-negative woman has amniocentesis at 16 weeks. Is Anti-D required?
5. A Rh D-negative woman with an ectopic pregnancy receives methotrexate. Is Anti-D prophylaxis indicated?

EMQ47: Dosage of Anti-D Prophylaxis

Options:

a) 250 IU

b) 500 IU

c) 1000 IU

d) 1500 IU

e) No Anti-D required

Questions:

1. A Rh D-negative woman undergoes amniocentesis at 18 weeks. What dosage of Anti-D is recommended?
2. A Rh D-negative woman experiences a spontaneous miscarriage at 10 weeks with heavy bleeding. What dosage of Anti-D should be administered?
3. A Rh D-negative woman at 32 weeks undergoes an external cephalic version. What is the appropriate dosage of Anti-D?
4. A Rh D-negative woman undergoes an elective abortion at 9 weeks gestation. What dosage of Anti-D is indicated?

5. A Rh D-negative woman delivers via cesarean section at 39 weeks. What dosage of Anti-D should she receive?

EMQ48: Management of Delayed Anti-D Administration

Options:

a) Administer within 10 days

b) Repeat dose after 24 hours

c) Monitor antibody levels only

d) No further action required

e) Administer higher dose

Questions:

1. A Rh D-negative woman receives Anti-D 5 days after a potentially sensitising event. What should be done next?
2. A Rh D-negative woman has a traumatic delivery and receives Anti-D after 9 days. What is the next step?
3. A Rh D-negative woman receives a lower dose of Anti-D than required for her gestational age. What should be done?
4. Anti-D was administered 11 days after a significant trauma in a Rh D-negative woman. What is the appropriate action?
5. A Rh D-negative woman receives Anti-D 2 days after amniocentesis. What further management is required?

EMQ49: Potentially Sensitising Events Requiring Anti-D Prophylaxis

Options:

a) First trimester miscarriage with bleeding

b) Antepartum haemorrhage at 22 weeks

c) Ectopic pregnancy treated surgically

d) Spontaneous rupture of membranes at term

e) Therapeutic abortion at 8 weeks

Questions:

1. A Rh D-negative woman experiences antepartum haemorrhage at 22 weeks. Does this event require Anti-D prophylaxis?
2. A Rh D-negative woman undergoes surgical management for an ectopic pregnancy. Is Anti-D prophylaxis required?
3. A Rh D-negative woman has a spontaneous rupture of membranes at term. Should Anti-D be given?
4. A Rh D-negative woman undergoes a therapeutic abortion at 8 weeks gestation. Should she receive Anti-D?
5. A Rh D-negative woman has a first-trimester miscarriage at 8 weeks with moderate bleeding. Is Anti-D needed?

EMQ50: Management of Anti-D in Special Cases

Options:

a) No further action needed

b) Administer Anti-D within 72 hours

c) Administer Anti-D within 10 days

d) Repeat Kleihauer-Betke test

e) Perform antibody titre monitoring

Questions:

1. A Rh D-negative woman receives Anti-D 7 days after an external cephalic version. What is the appropriate management?
2. A Rh D-negative woman who underwent cesarean section receives Anti-D after 5 days. What should be done?
3. After a traumatic delivery, a Rh D-negative woman receives Anti-D 4 days later. What is the appropriate next step?
4. A Rh D-negative woman undergoes therapeutic abortion and receives Anti-D 6 days later. What is the appropriate management?
5. A Rh D-negative woman experiences minor trauma at 28 weeks gestation and receives Anti-D within 72 hours. What is the appropriate action?

Recurrent Miscarriage

Definition and Epidemiology: Miscarriage refers to the spontaneous loss of a pregnancy before the fetus reaches viability, defined as before 24 weeks of gestation. Recurrent miscarriage is the loss of three or more consecutive pregnancies and affects approximately 1% of couples attempting to conceive. The risk of miscarriage increases with the number of prior miscarriages and is significantly influenced by maternal age, rising sharply after age 35.

Risk Factors:

- **Epidemiological Factors:** Maternal age (≥35 years) and paternal age (≥40 years) are key risk factors. Lifestyle factors, such as smoking, heavy alcohol consumption, and obesity, have also been associated with increased miscarriage risk. The risk increases with maternal age, with the highest risk (93%) in women aged ≥45 years.

- **Genetic/Chromosomal Factors:** Chromosomal anomalies are found in 3-5% of couples with recurrent miscarriage, with the most common being balanced translocations. Embryonic chromosomal abnormalities account for 30-57% of recurrent miscarriages. Parental karyotyping is recommended if chromosomal abnormalities are detected in the products of conception.

- **Uterine Structural Anomalies:** Structural anomalies of the uterus are reported in 1.8-37.6% of women with recurrent miscarriage. However, the role of surgical correction in preventing further miscarriages remains uncertain, and the risks of such surgeries, including infertility and adhesions, must be considered.

- **Cervical Weakness:** Cervical weakness, a cause of second-trimester miscarriages, is difficult to diagnose and is typically based on clinical history. Cervical cerclage may be beneficial for women with a history of second-trimester miscarriage and a short cervix detected via transvaginal ultrasound before 24 weeks of gestation.

- **Thrombophilia:** Both inherited and acquired thrombophilias, such as antiphospholipid syndrome, have been linked to recurrent miscarriage. Antiphospholipid syndrome, in particular, is a significant and treatable cause, with treatment involving aspirin and heparin significantly improving live birth rates.

Investigations and Management:

- **Investigations:** Key investigations for recurrent miscarriage include testing for antiphospholipid antibodies, pelvic ultrasound, and cytogenetic analysis of the products of conception. Parental karyotyping may be warranted if abnormalities are detected.

- **Management:** Women with unexplained recurrent miscarriage have a good prognosis for future pregnancies, especially with supportive care in dedicated early pregnancy assessment units. Psychological support and attendance at specialized clinics may also have a positive impact, although this has not been extensively studied.

Supportive Care:

- **Unexplained Recurrent Miscarriage:** Women with unexplained recurrent miscarriage may have a successful pregnancy outcome in approximately 75% of cases when provided with supportive care alone. The prognosis is less favourable with increasing maternal age and the number of previous miscarriages. Psychological support and consistent monitoring in early pregnancy clinics are recommended, though more research is needed to fully understand their benefits.

Single Best Answer Questions:

SBA 141:
A 37-year-old woman presents with a history of three consecutive first-trimester miscarriages. What is the most significant risk factor in this case?
a) Smoking
b) Obesity
c) Maternal age
d) Polycystic ovary syndrome (PCOS)
e) Low folate levels

SBA 142:
In women over 40 years of age, what is the approximate risk of miscarriage in the first trimester?
a) 20%
b) 25%
c) 40%
d) 50%
e) 75%

SBA 143:
A couple presents with a history of recurrent miscarriage. The female partner is 30 years old, and the male partner is 46 years old. Which factor is most likely contributing to the recurrent miscarriage?
a) Female partner's age
b) Male partner's age
c) Obesity
d) Smoking
e) Hypertension

SBA 144:
Which uterine abnormality is most commonly associated

with an increased risk of recurrent miscarriage?
a) Bicornuate uterus
b) Septate uterus
c) Unicornuate uterus
d) Didelphic uterus
e) Arcuate uterus

SBA 145:
What percentage of women with recurrent miscarriage will have a chromosomal abnormality detected in the products of conception?
a) 5-10%
b) 15-20%
c) 30-57%
d) 60-70%
e) 80-90%

SBA 146:
Which of the following thrombophilias is most strongly associated with an increased risk of recurrent miscarriage?
a) Protein S deficiency
b) Factor V Leiden mutation
c) Antiphospholipid syndrome
d) Prothrombin gene mutation
e) Antithrombin III deficiency

SBA 147:
A 28-year-old woman with a history of three consecutive first-trimester miscarriages undergoes investigations. Which initial investigation should be performed to identify potential causes of recurrent miscarriage?
a) Thyroid function tests
b) Antiphospholipid antibody testing

c) Pelvic ultrasound
d) Glucose tolerance test
e) TORCH screen

SBA 148:
What is the recommended management for a woman with a history of recurrent miscarriage and a confirmed septate uterus?
a) No treatment
b) Hysteroscopic resection of the septum
c) Abdominal myomectomy
d) Progesterone supplementation
e) Cervical cerclage

SBA 149:
A 32-year-old woman with a history of two second-trimester miscarriages is suspected to have cervical insufficiency. Which of the following is the best management option?
a) Bed rest throughout pregnancy
b) Progesterone supplementation
c) Serial cervical length monitoring with cerclage if needed
d) Immediate cervical cerclage in the first trimester
e) Daily aspirin

SBA 150:
A 30-year-old woman presents with three consecutive first-trimester miscarriages and normal parental karyotyping. What is the most appropriate next step in her management?
a) IVF with preimplantation genetic diagnosis
b) Referral for a hysterosalpingogram
c) Thrombophilia screen

d) Empirical treatment with low-dose aspirin
e) Reassurance and expectant management

SBA 151:
In a woman with a history of recurrent miscarriage and diagnosed antiphospholipid syndrome, what is the recommended first-line treatment during pregnancy?
a) Aspirin alone
b) Aspirin and low-molecular-weight heparin (LMWH)
c) Low-molecular-weight heparin (LMWH) alone
d) Prednisolone
e) Intravenous immunoglobulin (IVIG)

SBA 152:
What is the approximate success rate for a subsequent pregnancy in women with unexplained recurrent miscarriage who receive supportive care alone?
a) 30%
b) 50%
c) 75%
d) 90%
e) 95%

SBA 153:
A 35-year-old woman with a history of recurrent miscarriage is found to have a balanced translocation. Which of the following is the best management option?
a) Referral for preimplantation genetic diagnosis
b) Cervical cerclage
c) Empirical progesterone treatment
d) Hysteroscopic septum resection
e) Serial β-hCG monitoring

SBA 154:
Which of the following is the most common chromosomal abnormality identified in the products of conception in cases of recurrent miscarriage?
a) Trisomy 21
b) Turner syndrome
c) Trisomy 16
d) Klinefelter syndrome
e) Robertsonian translocation

SBA 155:
A 34-year-old woman with a history of three first-trimester miscarriages is found to have antiphospholipid antibodies. Which of the following is the most appropriate management for her next pregnancy?
a) Low-dose aspirin alone
b) Low-dose aspirin and low-molecular-weight heparin
c) High-dose aspirin alone
d) Steroids and intravenous immunoglobulin
e) Bed rest throughout pregnancy

SBA 156:
In a woman with recurrent miscarriage and a history of antiphospholipid syndrome, what is the most appropriate time to start low-molecular-weight heparin (LMWH) therapy during pregnancy?
a) Before conception
b) As soon as pregnancy is confirmed
c) At 12 weeks of gestation
d) At 20 weeks of gestation
e) After the first miscarriage

SBA 157:
What is the estimated risk of miscarriage in women aged

45 years or older?
a) 25%
b) 50%
c) 60%
d) 75%
e) 93%

SBA 158:
A 33-year-old woman with a history of recurrent miscarriage has undergone a series of investigations, all of which returned normal results. Which of the following is the best next step?
a) Empirical treatment with progesterone
b) Referral for IVF with genetic screening
c) Reassurance and expectant management
d) Surgical correction of uterine anomalies
e) Daily aspirin therapy

SBA 159:
In women with recurrent miscarriage and normal parental karyotypes, which genetic condition is most commonly found in the products of conception?
a) Turner syndrome
b) Down syndrome
c) Trisomy 16
d) Klinefelter syndrome
e) Patau syndrome

SBA 160:
What is the first-line treatment for recurrent miscarriage in women with antiphospholipid syndrome?
a) Intravenous immunoglobulin
b) Corticosteroids
c) Low-dose aspirin and low-molecular-weight heparin

d) High-dose aspirin
e) Empirical progesterone treatment

Extended Match Questions (EMQ)

EMQ 51: Investigations in Recurrent Miscarriage

Options: a) Parental karyotyping
b) Pelvic ultrasound scan
c) Testing for antiphospholipid antibodies
d) Testing for inherited thrombophilias
e) Hysteroscopy
f) TORCH screening

Questions:

1. A 26-year-old woman presents after three consecutive first-trimester miscarriages. She has no significant past medical history, and previous products of conception were normal.

2. A 30-year-old woman with a history of recurrent miscarriage is found to have a uterine septum on pelvic ultrasound.

3. A 32-year-old woman with a history of three recurrent miscarriages has a normal pelvic ultrasound and no family history of thrombophilia. She tests positive for lupus anticoagulant.

4. A 29-year-old woman with two previous miscarriages has a partner with a known chromosomal translocation.

5. A 34-year-old woman with a history of three recurrent miscarriages and a normal pelvic ultrasound presents with a history of thrombosis.

EMQ 52: Management Options for Uterine Anomalies in Recurrent Miscarriage

Options: a) Expectant management
b) Hysteroscopic resection
c) Laparoscopic resection
d) Uterine artery embolisation
e) Cervical cerclage
f) Combined hysteroscopy and laparoscopy

Questions:

1. A 27-year-old woman with recurrent miscarriage is found to have a septate uterus on 3D ultrasound.

2. A 33-year-old woman with a history of recurrent second-trimester losses has a diagnosis of cervical incompetence.

3. A 30-year-old woman with a known uterine fibroid presents with recurrent miscarriage. The fibroid is large and submucosal.

4. A 28-year-old woman with recurrent first-trimester miscarriage has a diagnosis of bicornuate uterus on MRI.

5. A 35-year-old woman with a uterine septum has had two previous miscarriages and now desires surgical correction.

EMQ 53: Risk Factors for Recurrent Miscarriage

Options: a) Maternal age >35 years
b) Smoking
c) Chromosomal anomalies
d) Thrombophilia
e) Uterine structural anomalies
f) Obesity

Questions:

1. A 40-year-old woman presents with three consecutive miscarriages. Her first pregnancy was at 37 years old.

2. A 32-year-old woman has had three miscarriages. Her partner has been diagnosed with a balanced translocation.

3. A 29-year-old woman has a history of recurrent miscarriage and smokes 15 cigarettes per day.

4. A 34-year-old woman with recurrent miscarriage has a normal karyotype but is found to have uterine fibroids.

5. A 30-year-old woman with a BMI of 32 presents after her second miscarriage.

EMQ 54: Prognostic Factors in Recurrent Miscarriage

Options: a) Presence of antiphospholipid antibodies
b) History of a previous live birth
c) Normal parental karyotype
d) Recurrent miscarriage without identified cause
e) Increasing maternal age
f) Presence of uterine anomaly

Questions:

1. A 38-year-old woman with a history of three consecutive miscarriages is found to have a normal pelvic ultrasound but tests positive for antiphospholipid antibodies.

2. A 35-year-old woman with recurrent miscarriage has previously delivered a healthy child at term.

3. A 32-year-old woman with a normal karyotype and no identified risk factors for miscarriage.

4. A 34-year-old woman with recurrent miscarriage and a known uterine septum.

5. A 42-year-old woman presents with a history of three consecutive miscarriages and a normal workup.

EMQ 55: Thrombophilia and Recurrent Miscarriage

Options: a) Factor V Leiden mutation
b) Prothrombin gene mutation
c) Antiphospholipid syndrome
d) Protein S deficiency
e) Protein C deficiency
f) Antithrombin III deficiency

Questions:

1. A 28-year-old woman with recurrent miscarriage tests positive for lupus anticoagulant and anticardiolipin antibodies.

2. A 31-year-old woman with recurrent miscarriage has a family history of venous thromboembolism and tests positive for Factor V Leiden mutation.

3. A 35-year-old woman with recurrent miscarriage has low protein S levels on thrombophilia screening.

4. A 29-year-old woman with recurrent miscarriage tests positive for the prothrombin gene mutation.

5. A 33-year-old woman with a history of recurrent miscarriage tests positive for antithrombin III deficiency.

EMQ 56: Causes of Second-Trimester Miscarriage in Recurrent Pregnancy Loss

Options: a) Cervical incompetence
b) Uterine fibroids
c) Antiphospholipid syndrome
d) Chromosomal abnormalities
e) Septate uterus
f) Progesterone deficiency

Questions:

1. A 30-year-old woman with three second-trimester losses presents with painless cervical dilation at 18 weeks during her most recent pregnancy.

2. A 34-year-old woman with recurrent second-trimester miscarriages is found to have a large submucosal fibroid on ultrasound.

3. A 29-year-old woman with a history of recurrent first-trimester miscarriages tests positive for lupus anticoagulant.

4. A 32-year-old woman with recurrent second-trimester losses is diagnosed with a uterine anomaly on hysteroscopy.

5. A 31-year-old woman with a history of recurrent miscarriage has an abnormal karyotype analysis of the products of conception from her last pregnancy.

EMQ 57: Management of Cervical Incompetence in Recurrent Miscarriage

Options: a) Cervical cerclage
b) Progesterone supplementation
c) Expectant management
d) Bed rest
e) Hysteroscopic resection
f) Laparoscopic resection

Questions:

1. A 28-year-old woman with a history of three second-trimester miscarriages and ultrasound evidence of cervical shortening.

2. A 30-year-old woman with a history of preterm birth and recurrent miscarriage, presenting with a short cervix detected on transvaginal ultrasound at 16 weeks.

3. A 32-year-old woman with a history of second-trimester loss and normal cervical length, presenting with recurrent miscarriage.

4. A 34-year-old woman with a history of second-trimester miscarriage, who has not benefited from previous cervical cerclage.

5. A 29-year-old woman with a history of recurrent miscarriages and a uterine septum diagnosed via hysteroscopy.

EMQ 58: Genetic Investigations in Recurrent Miscarriage

Options: a) Parental karyotyping
b) Genetic counselling
c) Preimplantation genetic diagnosis (PGD)
d) Cytogenetic analysis of products of conception
e) TORCH screening
f) Testing for Factor V Leiden mutation

Questions:

1. A 33-year-old woman with recurrent miscarriages and a partner with a balanced translocation.

2. A 28-year-old woman with a history of recurrent miscarriage and normal parental karyotypes, with

abnormal cytogenetic analysis of the last miscarriage.

3. A 32-year-old woman with three first-trimester miscarriages, with no known genetic abnormalities in either parent.

4. A 35-year-old woman with recurrent miscarriage and no identifiable genetic cause, seeking advice for future pregnancies.

5. A 29-year-old woman with a known history of recurrent miscarriage and suspected thrombophilia.

EMQ 59: Supportive Care in Recurrent Miscarriage

Options: a) Early pregnancy assessment unit (EPAU)
b) Psychological support
c) Aspirin and heparin therapy
d) Cervical cerclage
e) Bed rest
f) Expectant management

Questions:

1. A 31-year-old woman with recurrent miscarriage and no identified cause, seeking care in a specialized clinic.

2. A 34-year-old woman with antiphospholipid syndrome and a history of recurrent miscarriage.

3. A 29-year-old woman with recurrent second-trimester losses and a diagnosis of cervical incompetence.

4. A 32-year-old woman with recurrent miscarriage and significant anxiety about her current pregnancy.

5. A 30-year-old woman with recurrent first-trimester miscarriages, and normal investigations, seeking advice on management.

EMQ 60: Hormonal Factors in Recurrent Miscarriage

Options: a) Progesterone deficiency
b) Polycystic Ovary Syndrome (PCOS)
c) Thyroid dysfunction
d) Hyperprolactinemia
e) Ovarian insufficiency
f) Luteal phase defect

Questions:

1. A 30-year-old woman with recurrent first-trimester miscarriages and a history of irregular menstrual cycles, diagnosed with elevated prolactin levels.

2. A 32-year-old woman with a history of recurrent miscarriage, found to have low progesterone levels in the luteal phase.

3. A 29-year-old woman with recurrent miscarriage and a history of hypothyroidism.

4. A 28-year-old woman with a history of recurrent first-trimester miscarriages and a diagnosis of PCOS.

5. A 34-year-old woman with a history of recurrent miscarriage and reduced ovarian reserve.

Nausea and Vomiting in Pregnancy NVP, and Hyperemesis Gravidarum (HG)

Prevalence and Severity:

- NVP affects up to 90% of pregnant women.

- HG, a severe form of NVP, affects between 0.3% and 3.6% of pregnancies.

- The major mechanism of NVP and HG is related to hypersensitivity to growth differentiation factor-15 (GDF15), which causes symptoms like loss of appetite, nausea, vomiting, and weight loss.

- Genetic variants associated with GDF15 are the greatest genetic risk factor for HG and its recurrence.

Definition and Diagnosis:

- NVP is diagnosed when symptoms start before 16 weeks of gestation, excluding other causes.

- HG is diagnosed when symptoms are severe enough to cause an inability to eat, drink normally, and limit daily activities, with signs of dehydration.

- The Pregnancy-Unique Quantification of Emesis (PUQE) and HyperEmesis Level Prediction (HELP) tools can be used to classify and monitor the severity of NVP and HG.

- Ketonuria is not a reliable indicator of dehydration in pregnancy.

Clinical Presentation:

- NVP typically starts between 4th and 7th weeks of gestation, peaks around the 9th week, and resolves by the 20th week in 90% of women.
- HG may present with abnormal thyroid function tests, which usually resolve as the condition improves. Abnormal liver function tests are also common in up to 40% of women with HG.

Care and Management:

- Women with mild NVP can be managed in the community with antiemetics.
- Inpatient care is necessary for those with severe symptoms, clinical dehydration, weight loss, or when comorbidities are present.
- A combination of different antiemetics should be used for those who do not respond to a single treatment.
- First-line treatments include H1 histamines, phenothiazines, and pyridoxine-doxylamine.
- Second-line treatments include ondansetron and metoclopramide, with considerations for their safety and duration of use.
- Corticosteroids are reserved for cases where standard therapies have been ineffective.

Nutritional Support and Risks:

- Women with severe vomiting or reduced dietary intake should receive thiamine supplementation, particularly before administering dextrose or parenteral nutrition.

- Thromboprophylaxis should be considered for women admitted with HG, with low-molecular-weight heparin being the preferred option.
- Avoiding iron supplements may alleviate NVP symptoms in some women.

Antenatal Care:

- Discharge criteria include toleration of antiemetics, adequate oral nutrition and hydration, and management of concurrent conditions.
- Serial scans should be offered for fetal growth monitoring in women with persistent symptoms into late pregnancy.
- HG is associated with risks of low birth weight, small-for-gestational-age babies, and increased need for resuscitation or intensive care.

Rehydration and Nutrition:

- Normal saline with potassium chloride is recommended for intravenous hydration.
- Dextrose infusions are not recommended for fluid replacement in NVP and HG.
- Enteral and parenteral nutrition should be considered only when other treatments have failed, and with multidisciplinary support due to associated risks.

Psychosocial Impact and Long-Term Effects:

- HG can severely impact a woman's quality of life and mental health, with increased risks of postnatal depression (PND), anxiety, and PTSD.
- Women should receive psychological support if needed and be monitored for any persistent symptoms postnatally.
- Pre-emptive use of antiemetics and lifestyle modifications may reduce the risk of recurrence in future pregnancies.

Termination of Pregnancy:

- All therapeutic measures should be offered before considering termination.
- Termination of pregnancy is considered in severe, refractory cases where all treatments have failed.

Single Best Answer Questions:

SBA 161: What percentage of pregnant women are affected by Nausea and Vomiting in Pregnancy (NVP)?

a) 10%
b) 30%
c) 50%
d) 70%
e) 90%

SBA 162: What is the most likely diagnosis for a pregnant woman presenting with severe nausea, vomiting, weight loss, and dehydration?

a) Gastroenteritis
b) Hyperemesis gravidarum
c) Pyelonephritis
d) Migraine
e) Cholecystitis

SBA 163: Which genetic factor is most strongly associated with Hyperemesis Gravidarum (HG)?

a) BRCA1 mutation
b) GDF15 variants
c) CFTR mutation
d) FMR1 premutation
e) HLA-B27

SBA 164: At what gestational age does Nausea and Vomiting in Pregnancy (NVP) typically peak?

a) 5 weeks
b) 7 weeks

c) 9 weeks
d) 12 weeks
e) 14 weeks

SBA 165: Which of the following is NOT a first-line treatment for NVP?

a) H1 histamines
b) Phenothiazines
c) Pyridoxine-doxylamine
d) Ondansetron
e) Metoclopramide

SBA 166: Which clinical finding is most consistent with a diagnosis of Hyperemesis Gravidarum (HG)?

a) Presence of ketonuria
b) Elevated thyroid function tests
c) Elevated liver enzymes
d) Persistent vomiting causing weight loss and dehydration
e) All of the above

SBA 167: Which treatment is recommended as a second-line therapy for Hyperemesis Gravidarum?

a) H1 histamines
b) Pyridoxine-doxylamine
c) Ondansetron
d) Antacids
e) Ginger supplements

SBA 168: What is the recommended action if a woman with Hyperemesis Gravidarum does not respond to standard antiemetic therapies?

a) Discontinue all treatment
b) Use corticosteroids
c) Increase hydration only
d) Initiate high-dose vitamin supplements
e) Offer immediate termination of pregnancy

SBA 169: What should be included in the management plan for a woman with severe Hyperemesis Gravidarum who requires hospital admission?

a) Normal saline with potassium chloride for hydration
b) Dextrose infusions for energy
c) High doses of iron supplements
d) Initiate broad-spectrum antibiotics
e) Immediate enteral nutrition

SBA 170: What percentage of pregnancies are affected by Hyperemesis Gravidarum (HG)?

a) 0.1%
b) 0.5%
c) 1.0%
d) 2.5%
e) 3.6%

SBA 171: In Hyperemesis Gravidarum, which factor is not typically a reliable indicator of dehydration?

a) Blood pressure
b) Heart rate
c) Serum electrolytes

d) Ketonuria
e) Urine output

SBA 172: What nutritional support should be given to women with severe vomiting or reduced dietary intake in Hyperemesis Gravidarum?

a) Thiamine supplementation
b) High-calcium supplements
c) Increased protein intake
d) Iron supplements
e) Folic acid only

SBA 173: What potential complication is associated with Hyperemesis Gravidarum during pregnancy?

a) Increased risk of preterm labour
b) Increased risk of stillbirth
c) Small-for-gestational-age babies
d) Macrosomia
e) Gestational diabetes

SBA 174: Which statement is true regarding the psychosocial impact of Hyperemesis Gravidarum?

a) It has no long-term effects
b) It is linked with increased risks of postnatal depression
c) It does not affect the quality of life
d) It only affects mental health during pregnancy
e) It is linked with increased risks of pre-eclampsia

SBA 175: Which statement is correct regarding the use of ondansetron in the treatment of Hyperemesis Gravidarum?

a) It is a first-line therapy
b) It is recommended for short-term use only due to safety concerns
c) It should be avoided in all pregnant women
d) It is safe for use throughout the entire pregnancy
e) It has no side effects

SBA 176: When should antiemetic treatment typically be stopped in a woman with Hyperemesis Gravidarum?

a) After 12 weeks of gestation
b) Once the symptoms improve and she can maintain oral intake
c) Immediately after admission to the hospital
d) At 20 weeks of gestation
e) After delivery

SBA 177: What is the first-line treatment for mild Nausea and Vomiting in Pregnancy (NVP) managed in the community?

a) Pyridoxine-doxylamine
b) Antacids
c) Ondansetron
d) Corticosteroids
e) Vitamin B12 supplements

SBA 178: In which scenario is hospitalization most likely required for a woman with NVP or HG?

a) Mild nausea with occasional vomiting
b) Persistent vomiting with significant weight loss and dehydration
c) Slight aversion to certain foods
d) Morning sickness that is well-controlled with over-the-

counter remedies
e) Fatigue without vomiting

SBA 179: Which of the following is a common complication of Hyperemesis Gravidarum?

a) Hypothyroidism
b) Preterm labour
c) Electrolyte imbalances
d) Hypertension
e) Diabetes mellitus

SBA 180: In the context of Hyperemesis Gravidarum, which investigation is least likely to be informative?

a) Serum electrolytes
b) Liver function tests
c) Thyroid function tests
d) Full blood count
e) Blood cultures

SBA 181: What is the most common gestational age range for the onset of nausea and vomiting in pregnancy (NVP)?

a) 2–4 weeks
b) 4–7 weeks
c) 8–10 weeks
d) 11–14 weeks
e) After 14 weeks

SBA 182: What is the first-line pharmacological treatment for managing mild to moderate nausea and vomiting in pregnancy?

a) Metoclopramide
b) Ondansetron
c) Pyridoxine-doxylamine
d) Corticosteroids
e) Domperidone

SBA 183: What is the primary concern for a pregnant woman presenting with Hyperemesis Gravidarum and ketonuria?

a) Anaemia
b) Dehydration
c) Hyperthyroidism
d) Hypoglycaemia
e) Infection

SBA 184: Which of the following is a common abnormal laboratory finding in Hyperemesis Gravidarum?

a) Hypercalcaemia
b) Hypokalaemia
c) Hyperglycaemia
d) Hyponatraemia
e) Hyperbilirubinaemia

SBA 185: Which antiemetic is generally reserved for use when first-line treatments fail in the management of Hyperemesis Gravidarum?

a) Ondansetron
b) Cyclizine
c) Promethazine
d) Metoclopramide
e) Prochlorperazine

SBA 186: What is the recommended intravenous fluid for rehydration in patients with Hyperemesis Gravidarum?

a) Dextrose 5%
b) Normal saline with potassium chloride
c) Hartmann's solution
d) Albumin
e) Dextrose 10%

SBA 187: Which of the following is a potential long-term effect of Hyperemesis Gravidarum if left untreated?

a) Chronic hypertension
b) Gestational diabetes
c) Post-traumatic stress disorder (PTSD)
d) Preterm labour
e) Preeclampsia

SBA 188: What is the key diagnostic tool for assessing the severity of nausea and vomiting in pregnancy?

a) Blood glucose monitoring
b) Pelvic ultrasound
c) Pregnancy-Unique Quantification of Emesis (PUQE) score
d) Serum β-hCG levels
e) Complete blood count

SBA 189: What is the risk factor most strongly associated with the recurrence of Hyperemesis Gravidarum in subsequent pregnancies?

a) High body mass index (BMI)
b) Multiple gestation
c) Previous history of Hyperemesis Gravidarum

d) Low socioeconomic status
e) Smoking

SBA 190: What is the preferred approach for managing a patient with mild nausea and vomiting in pregnancy who prefers not to take medications?

a) Admission for intravenous fluids
b) Ginger supplements
c) Antiemetic therapy
d) Hospitalization for observation
e) Discharge with no intervention

SBA 191: At what gestational age does Hyperemesis Gravidarum most commonly resolve in affected women?

a) 8 weeks
b) 12 weeks
c) 16 weeks
d) 20 weeks
e) 24 weeks

SBA 192: Which of the following complications is least likely to be associated with Hyperemesis Gravidarum?

a) Electrolyte imbalances
b) Significant weight loss
c) Low birth weight
d) Fetal macrosomia
e) Nutritional deficiencies

SBA 193: In cases of severe Hyperemesis Gravidarum, which of the following is the most appropriate next step after initial stabilization?

a) Immediate discharge
b) Outpatient follow-up in 1 week
c) Consideration of termination of pregnancy
d) Referral to a specialist or hospital admission
e) Prescription of iron supplements

SBA 194: What dietary modification is commonly recommended for women experiencing nausea and vomiting in pregnancy?

a) High-fat diet
b) Small, frequent meals
c) High-protein, low-carbohydrate diet
d) Fasting for 12 hours
e) High-fibre diet

SBA 195: Which of the following is the least likely indicator of dehydration in a patient with Hyperemesis Gravidarum?

a) Hypotension
b) Tachycardia
c) Ketonuria
d) Dry mucous membranes
e) Decreased urine output

SBA 196: When should parenteral nutrition be considered for a patient with Hyperemesis Gravidarum?

a) After 1 week of symptoms
b) When oral intake is severely limited and other treatments have failed
c) As the first-line treatment
d) When weight gain is normal
e) In the first trimester

SBA 197: What is the purpose of administering thiamine supplementation in patients with Hyperemesis Gravidarum?

a) To prevent neural tube defects
b) To manage gestational diabetes
c) To prevent Wernicke's encephalopathy
d) To enhance fetal growth
e) To reduce nausea

SBA 198: What psychological condition is most commonly associated with severe cases of Hyperemesis Gravidarum?

a) Postnatal depression
b) Anxiety
c) Schizophrenia
d) Bipolar disorder
e) Obsessive-compulsive disorder

SBA 199: Which of the following is least likely to be part of the discharge criteria for a patient hospitalized with Hyperemesis Gravidarum?

a) Ability to tolerate oral fluids
b) Significant weight loss
c) Stabilized electrolytes
d) Controlled nausea with antiemetics
e) Adequate hydration status

SBA 200: In what percentage of pregnancies does Hyperemesis Gravidarum occur?

a) 0.1%
b) 0.3%
c) 1.0%
d) 2.5%
e) 5.0%

Extended Match Questions (EMQ)

EMQ 61: Diagnosis of Nausea and Vomiting in Pregnancy (NVP) and Hyperemesis Gravidarum (HG)

Options:

a) Mild NVP
b) Moderate NVP
c) Hyperemesis Gravidarum
d) Gastroenteritis
e) Dehydration

Questions:

1. A 24-year-old woman at 7 weeks of gestation presents with mild nausea in the morning, but no vomiting. She can tolerate small meals throughout the day.

2. A 28-year-old woman at 9 weeks of gestation reports constant nausea with frequent vomiting, leading to difficulty in performing daily activities and a 5% loss of body weight.

3. A 30-year-old woman at 10 weeks of gestation presents with severe nausea, vomiting multiple times daily, significant weight loss, and signs of dehydration.

4. A 26-year-old woman at 8 weeks of gestation has mild nausea and vomiting that occurs 1-2 times daily, but she can manage most of her routine activities.

5. A 22-year-old woman presents with severe vomiting, diarrhoea, abdominal pain, and fever, which started suddenly two days ago.

EMQ 62: Management Options for NVP and HG

Options:

a) Reassurance and dietary advice
b) Antiemetic therapy
c) Hospital admission with intravenous fluids
d) Nutritional support with enteral feeding
e) Referral for psychiatric support

Questions:

1. A 25-year-old woman at 6 weeks of gestation experiences mild nausea and occasional vomiting. She is able to maintain oral intake and hydration.

2. A 30-year-old woman at 9 weeks of gestation with severe nausea and vomiting is unable to keep down fluids or food and shows signs of dehydration.

3. A 28-year-old woman at 8 weeks of gestation presents with persistent nausea and vomiting unresponsive to initial antiemetics, leading to significant weight loss.

4. A 32-year-old woman with Hyperemesis Gravidarum reports symptoms of depression and anxiety.

5. A 27-year-old woman at 7 weeks of gestation experiences moderate nausea and vomiting, managed with small frequent meals and oral hydration, but she is struggling with routine tasks.

EMQ 63: Risk Factors for Hyperemesis Gravidarum

Options:

a) Nulliparity
b) Twin pregnancy
c) History of HG in previous pregnancy
d) Obesity
e) Low socioeconomic status

Questions:

1. A 29-year-old woman at 8 weeks of gestation presents with severe vomiting and has a history of similar symptoms in her last pregnancy.

2. A 30-year-old woman at 7 weeks of gestation is diagnosed with Hyperemesis Gravidarum and is currently carrying twins.

3. A 25-year-old woman at 9 weeks of gestation is experiencing mild NVP. This is her first pregnancy.

4. A 32-year-old woman at 6 weeks of gestation with a BMI of 35 reports moderate nausea and vomiting.

5. A 28-year-old woman living in a low-income area presents with severe vomiting and dehydration at 10 weeks of gestation.

EMQ 64: Complications of Hyperemesis Gravidarum

Options:

a) Electrolyte imbalance
b) Fetal growth restriction
c) Preterm delivery
d) Postnatal depression
e) Gestational diabetes

Questions:

1. A 31-year-old woman with severe Hyperemesis Gravidarum at 18 weeks of gestation is diagnosed with hyponatremia and hypokalemia.

2. A 28-year-old woman with a history of Hyperemesis Gravidarum during pregnancy delivers a baby at 36 weeks with a birth weight below the 10th percentile.

3. A 26-year-old woman at 34 weeks of gestation presents with preterm labour after a pregnancy complicated by Hyperemesis Gravidarum.

4. A 30-year-old woman who experienced severe Hyperemesis Gravidarum reports symptoms of anxiety and depression two months after delivery.

5. A 32-year-old woman with HG at 14 weeks of gestation is diagnosed with a condition that usually manifests in the third trimester and is associated with insulin resistance.

EMQ 65: Investigations in NVP and HG

Options:

a) Serum electrolytes
b) Thyroid function tests
c) Liver function tests
d) Ultrasound scan
e) Urinalysis for ketones

Questions:

1. A 29-year-old woman at 10 weeks of gestation with Hyperemesis Gravidarum presents with jaundice and elevated liver enzymes.

2. A 26-year-old woman at 8 weeks of gestation with severe vomiting and weight loss is found to have low potassium levels.

3. A 32-year-old woman with persistent nausea and vomiting has a family history of thyroid disease. Blood tests show elevated thyroid-stimulating hormone (TSH).

4. A 28-year-old woman at 12 weeks of gestation presents with persistent nausea, vomiting, and weight loss. An ultrasound scan is performed to rule out a molar pregnancy.

5. A 27-year-old woman at 7 weeks of gestation with moderate nausea and vomiting has a urinalysis showing +2 ketones, raising concerns about dehydration.

EMQ 66: Differential Diagnosis of Nausea and Vomiting in Pregnancy (NVP)

Options:

a) Hyperemesis Gravidarum
b) Gastroenteritis
c) Pyelonephritis
d) Molar pregnancy
e) Gallstones

Questions:

1. A 26-year-old woman at 10 weeks of gestation presents with severe nausea and vomiting,

weight loss, and a fundal height larger than expected for dates.

2. A 28-year-old woman at 8 weeks of gestation complains of nausea, vomiting, fever, and dysuria. Urinalysis reveals significant bacteriuria.

3. A 30-year-old woman at 9 weeks of gestation presents with severe nausea and vomiting, and laboratory results show elevated liver enzymes and right upper quadrant pain.

4. A 27-year-old woman at 12 weeks of gestation experiences persistent vomiting and vaginal bleeding. An ultrasound scan reveals the absence of a fetal heartbeat and the presence of an abnormal mass.

5. A 24-year-old woman at 7 weeks of gestation presents with sudden onset of nausea, vomiting, and diarrhoea after consuming food from a restaurant.

EMQ 67: Management of Hyperemesis Gravidarum

Options:

a) Oral rehydration therapy
b) Intravenous fluid replacement
c) Hospital admission
d) Thiamine supplementation
e) Termination of pregnancy

Questions:

1. A 29-year-old woman at 9 weeks of gestation presents with severe dehydration and persistent vomiting despite oral antiemetics.

2. A 30-year-old woman at 7 weeks of gestation is unable to maintain hydration and nutrition due to excessive vomiting and weight loss.

3. A 32-year-old woman with HG at 10 weeks of gestation is at risk of Wernicke's encephalopathy due to prolonged vomiting and poor nutritional intake.

4. A 28-year-old woman at 8 weeks of gestation experiences mild nausea and vomiting, which improves with dietary modifications and oral hydration.

5. A 35-year-old woman with severe, refractory HG at 14 weeks of gestation has not responded to multiple therapies and is considering her options.

EMQ 68: Risk Factors for NVP and HG

Options:

a) History of motion sickness
b) Twin pregnancy
c) Advanced maternal age
d) Female fetus
e) Family history of HG

Questions:

1. A 25-year-old woman at 8 weeks of gestation with a strong family history of HG presents with severe nausea and vomiting.

2. A 30-year-old woman at 10 weeks of gestation is carrying twins and experiences severe nausea and vomiting.

3. A 27-year-old woman with a history of motion sickness is 9 weeks pregnant and presents with moderate nausea and vomiting.

4. A 35-year-old woman at 7 weeks of gestation is experiencing mild nausea and vomiting. This is her first pregnancy.

5. A 29-year-old woman at 12 weeks of gestation has severe nausea and vomiting, and an ultrasound confirms a female fetus.

EMQ 69: Complications of Hyperemesis Gravidarum

Options:

a) Electrolyte imbalance
b) Wernicke's encephalopathy
c) Small for gestational age (SGA) infant
d) Post-traumatic stress disorder (PTSD)
e) Spontaneous abortion

Questions:

1. A 31-year-old woman at 14 weeks of gestation with severe HG presents with confusion, ataxia, and ophthalmoplegia.

2. A 28-year-old woman with a history of severe HG delivers a baby at 37 weeks with a birth weight below the 10th percentile.

3. A 26-year-old woman at 10 weeks of gestation with HG is found to have low potassium and sodium levels on blood tests.

4. A 30-year-old woman with HG develops anxiety and flashbacks related to her pregnancy experience.

5. A 27-year-old woman at 16 weeks of gestation with persistent HG has a spontaneous miscarriage.

EMQ 70: Long-Term Management of HG

Options:

a) Pre-emptive use of antiemetics
b) Lifestyle modifications
c) Psychological support
d) Nutritional counselling
e) Monitoring for postnatal depression

Questions:

1. A 28-year-old woman with a history of HG is planning another pregnancy and seeks advice on how to reduce the risk of recurrence.

2. A 30-year-old woman at 12 weeks of gestation with HG is concerned about the long-term impact on her mental health and requests support.

3. A 32-year-old woman at 10 weeks of gestation with HG is struggling to maintain adequate nutrition and requires dietary advice.

4. A 27-year-old woman at 14 weeks of gestation with HG has been admitted to the hospital multiple times and is advised to consider psychological support.

5. A 31-year-old woman with a history of HG and postnatal depression is being monitored closely during her current pregnancy to prevent a recurrence.

Answers

Single Best Answer (SBA): Answers

SBA 1:
Answer: c) Repeat serum hCG in 48 hours
Explanation: Serial serum hCG measurements help to monitor the progression of pregnancy, especially in cases of PUL where the location of the pregnancy is not visible on ultrasound.

SBA 2:
Answer: c) 6 weeks
Explanation: Early pregnancy assessment services should be available from around 6 weeks of gestation, as this is typically when early pregnancy complications can start to be detected.

SBA 3:
Answer: b) Positive pregnancy test but no pregnancy visible on scan
Explanation: This is the defining characteristic of a pregnancy of unknown location (PUL), where further investigation is needed to determine if the pregnancy is ectopic, intrauterine, or failing.

SBA 4:
Answer: b) 1500 IU/l
Explanation: A transvaginal ultrasound should be considered if the serum hCG level is 1500 IU/L or higher, as this is the threshold at which a pregnancy should generally be visible on the scan.

SBA 5:
Answer: c) To assess and manage early pregnancy complications
Explanation: The primary goal of early pregnancy assessment services is to manage complications such as pain, bleeding, and other issues that arise in the early stages of pregnancy.

SBA 6:
Answer: b) Accident & Emergency (A&E) department
Explanation: Women with severe symptoms should be referred to the nearest facility with access to specialist clinical assessment and ultrasound scanning, such as an A&E department.

SBA 7:
Answer: b) Women with a history of recurrent miscarriage, previous ectopic pregnancy, or molar pregnancy
Explanation: These women are at higher risk of complications and can self-refer to early pregnancy assessment services for prompt care.

SBA 8:
Answer: c) Immediate clinical review by a senior gynaecologist
Explanation: Worsening symptoms in a woman with PUL may indicate an ectopic pregnancy or another serious condition, requiring urgent clinical assessment.

SBA 9:
Answer: d) 14 days after the second serum hCG test
Explanation: If the test is negative, no further action is

required. If positive, the woman should return for a clinical review.

SBA 10

Answer: b) Discharge with routine antenatal care
Explanation: Once a viable intrauterine pregnancy is confirmed, there is no need for further emergency assessment. The woman can be reassured and discharged to continue routine antenatal care.

SBA 11

Answer: c) Clinical symptoms
Explanation: In the assessment of a pregnancy of unknown location (PUL), clinical symptoms such as pain and bleeding should take priority over serum hCG levels, as these can be more indicative of a potential ectopic pregnancy or other complications.

SBA 12

Answer: d) A pregnancy should be visible on ultrasound
Explanation: At hCG levels greater than 6000 mIU/mL, a pregnancy should typically be visible on an abdominal ultrasound. If no pregnancy is seen, further investigation is warranted to rule out ectopic pregnancy or other issues.

SBA 13

Answer: d) Within 72 hours
Explanation: Anti-D immunoglobulin should be administered within 72 hours of a potentially sensitising

event in a Rh D-negative woman to prevent alloimmunisation.

SBA 14

Answer: b) No further action needed
Explanation: If the urine pregnancy test is negative 14 days after the second hCG test, it indicates that the pregnancy has likely resolved, and no further follow-up is necessary.

SBA 15

Answer: b) Immediate clinical review for possible ectopic pregnancy
Explanation: Shoulder tip pain can be a sign of diaphragmatic irritation due to intra-abdominal bleeding, often associated with ectopic pregnancy, requiring urgent evaluation.

SBA 16

Answer: a) Self-referral to early pregnancy assessment service
Explanation: Women with a history of recurrent miscarriage can self-refer directly to early pregnancy assessment services for immediate care and monitoring.

SBA 17

Answer: a) No anti-D immunoglobulin needed
Explanation: Anti-D is not required for a Rh D-negative woman following a first-trimester miscarriage at 8 weeks if no surgical management was performed, as the risk of sensitisation is low.

SBA 18

Answer: d) Failing pregnancy of unknown location
Explanation: Stable hCG levels and the absence of symptoms in a woman with PUL suggest a failing pregnancy, which often resolves without further intervention.

SBA 19

Answer: d) Culdocentesis
Explanation: Culdocentesis is not routinely recommended in the management of PUL; the diagnosis is usually based on serial hCG levels, ultrasound, and clinical symptoms.

SBA 20

Answer: b) Repeat hCG in 48 hours
Explanation: When hCG levels are 2000 IU/L with no visible pregnancy, repeating hCG after 48 hours helps assess whether the pregnancy is progressing normally, which can guide further management decisions.

SBA 21
c) Ectopic pregnancy
Explanation: The presentation of lower abdominal pain, vaginal bleeding, and hemodynamic instability, along with an ultrasound showing free fluid in the pelvis, strongly suggests a ruptured ectopic pregnancy.

SBA 22
c) Methotrexate therapy
Explanation: The patient is hemodynamically stable with

a small ectopic mass and a serum hCG level below 5000 IU/L, making her a candidate for methotrexate therapy.

SBA 23
b) Methotrexate therapy
Explanation: The patient has a low hCG level and is stable, which makes her suitable for methotrexate therapy, especially given the history of tubal surgery.

SBA 24
d) Heterotopic pregnancy
Explanation: The combination of an intrauterine pregnancy with an adnexal mass, particularly following IVF, suggests a heterotopic pregnancy, where both intrauterine and ectopic pregnancies coexist.

SBA 25
d) Laparotomy
Explanation: The patient is hemodynamically unstable, indicating a possible ruptured ectopic pregnancy requiring emergency surgical intervention through laparotomy.

SBA 26
c) Repeat serum hCG in 48 hours
Explanation: An unclear ultrasound with an hCG level of 1500 IU/L suggests that repeating the hCG level in 48 hours can help confirm the diagnosis of an ectopic pregnancy or early intrauterine pregnancy.

SBA 27
b) Methotrexate therapy
Explanation: The patient's hCG level is below 5000 IU/L, and there is no intrauterine pregnancy with an adnexal mass, making methotrexate a suitable option.

SBA 28
b) Tubal pregnancy
Explanation: The clinical scenario strongly suggests a tubal pregnancy, which is the most common type of

ectopic pregnancy, especially with the absence of an intrauterine pregnancy on ultrasound.

SBA 29
c) Ectopic pregnancy
Explanation: The presence of lower abdominal pain, shoulder tip pain, and a positive pregnancy test without an intrauterine pregnancy is indicative of an ectopic pregnancy.

SBA 30
b) Laparotomy
Explanation: The patient is unstable with significant free fluid on ultrasound, indicating a ruptured ectopic pregnancy, requiring emergency surgical management through laparotomy.

SBA 31
d) Pregnancy of unknown location
Explanation: With an hCG level of 1200 IU/L and no visible pregnancy on ultrasound, the diagnosis is a pregnancy of unknown location, requiring close follow-up.

SBA 32
c) Repeat serum hCG in 48 hours
Explanation: Repeating the hCG level in 48 hours will help clarify the diagnosis, especially with an indeterminate ultrasound and hCG level.

SBA 33
c) Ruptured ectopic pregnancy
Explanation: The presentation of acute abdominal pain, vaginal bleeding, hypotension, and a large amount of free fluid strongly suggests a ruptured ectopic pregnancy.

SBA 34
b) Methotrexate therapy
Explanation: The patient is stable with a suitable hCG

level and an adnexal mass, making methotrexate therapy appropriate.

SBA 35
c) Laparoscopy
Explanation: With a high hCG level and no intrauterine pregnancy on ultrasound, along with an adnexal mass, laparoscopy is necessary to confirm and manage the ectopic pregnancy.

SBA 36
b) Ectopic pregnancy
Explanation: The presence of an adnexal mass and no intrauterine pregnancy on ultrasound in a woman with a history of pelvic inflammatory disease is highly indicative of an ectopic pregnancy.

SBA 37
b) Methotrexate therapy
Explanation: The patient is stable with an adnexal mass and hCG level that fits the criteria for methotrexate therapy.

SBA 38
b) Tubal pregnancy
Explanation: A gestational sac in the adnexa without an intrauterine pregnancy is most consistent with a tubal ectopic pregnancy.

SBA 39
b) Laparotomy
Explanation: The patient's unstable condition and significant free fluid on ultrasound suggest a ruptured ectopic pregnancy, requiring urgent laparotomy.

SBA 40
c) Ectopic pregnancy
Explanation: The presence of an adnexal mass, a high hCG level, and no intrauterine pregnancy points to an ectopic pregnancy.

SBA 41
c) Ectopic pregnancy
Explanation: The presence of an adnexal mass and no intrauterine pregnancy in a woman with a history of PID strongly suggests an ectopic pregnancy.

SBA 42
d) Emergency laparotomy
Explanation: Severe pain, hypotension, and free fluid on ultrasound in a woman with IVF indicate a likely ruptured ectopic pregnancy, necessitating urgent surgical intervention.

SBA 43
c) Ectopic pregnancy
Explanation: Shoulder tip pain, vaginal bleeding, and no intrauterine pregnancy on ultrasound with a positive hCG are classic signs of an ectopic pregnancy.

SBA 44
b) Repeat hCG in 48 hours
Explanation: With inconclusive ultrasound findings and low hCG, repeating hCG in 48 hours helps confirm or rule out ectopic pregnancy.

SBA 45
e) Emergency laparotomy
Explanation: Hemodynamic instability with a significant adnexal mass and free fluid suggests a ruptured ectopic pregnancy, requiring emergency laparotomy.

SBA 46
b) Methotrexate therapy
Explanation: The patient is stable with a small adnexal mass and hCG level suitable for methotrexate therapy.

SBA 47
c) Ruptured ectopic pregnancy
Explanation: The clinical presentation of severe pain,

hypotension, and free fluid in the abdomen is highly indicative of a ruptured ectopic pregnancy.

SBA 48
b) Methotrexate therapy
Explanation: A stable patient with a small adnexal mass and low hCG level is suitable for methotrexate therapy.

SBA 49
d) Laparoscopy
Explanation: The high hCG level and adnexal mass suggest an ectopic pregnancy, best managed with diagnostic and potentially therapeutic laparoscopy.

SBA 50
c) Ectopic pregnancy
Explanation: The presence of an adnexal mass and no intrauterine pregnancy on ultrasound with the clinical symptoms is indicative of an ectopic pregnancy.

SBA 51
c) Ectopic pregnancy
Explanation: The combination of an empty uterus, adnexal mass, and positive β-hCG in early pregnancy is highly suggestive of ectopic pregnancy.

SBA 52
b) 80%
Explanation: The majority of ectopic pregnancies occur in the ampullary section of the fallopian tube.

SBA 53
d) Laparotomy
Explanation: The clinical presentation suggests a ruptured ectopic pregnancy, requiring emergency surgical intervention.

SBA 54
c) Pelvic inflammatory disease
Explanation: PID is a well-known risk factor for ectopic pregnancy due to damage to the fallopian tubes.

SBA 55
b) 11
Explanation: The incidence of ectopic pregnancy in the UK is approximately 11 per 1000 pregnancies.

SBA 56
c) Diagnostic laparoscopy
Explanation: The presence of a complex adnexal mass in a symptomatic patient warrants surgical exploration.

SBA 57
e) Abdominal cavity
Explanation: Ectopic pregnancies are least common in the abdominal cavity compared to other locations.

SBA 58
b) Methotrexate therapy
Explanation: The patient is stable, with a low β-hCG and small adnexal mass, making her a candidate for methotrexate.

SBA 59
c) Extrauterine gestational sac with a yolk sac
Explanation: This ultrasound finding is a clear indicator of a tubal ectopic pregnancy.

SBA 60
c) 65–95%
Explanation: The success rate of single-dose methotrexate in ectopic pregnancies varies between 65% and 95%.

SBA 61
a) Ruptured ectopic pregnancy
Explanation: The presence of hypotension and free fluid in the abdomen strongly suggests a ruptured ectopic pregnancy.

SBA 62
c) Repeat β-hCG in 48 hours
Explanation: If ultrasound findings are inconclusive,

repeating β-hCG levels in 48 hours helps determine the viability and location of the pregnancy.

SBA 63
c) 3.2–5.0%
Explanation: The recurrence risk of a Caesarean section scar ectopic pregnancy is reported as 3.2–5.0%.

SBA 64
d) Laparoscopy
Explanation: The patient has a high β-hCG level and an adnexal mass, indicating the need for surgical management, often via laparoscopy.

SBA 65
c) Methotrexate therapy
Explanation: Methotrexate is appropriate for a stable patient with a small unruptured ectopic pregnancy and a β-hCG level less than 5000 IU/L.

SBA 66
d) Ampullary section of the fallopian tube
Explanation: The most common site for an ectopic pregnancy is the ampullary section of the fallopian tube.

SBA 67
b) Ectopic pregnancy
Explanation: The clinical presentation, combined with a positive pregnancy test and no intrauterine pregnancy on ultrasound, is highly suggestive of an ectopic pregnancy.

SBA 68
e) Hemoperitoneum on ultrasound
Explanation: The presence of hemoperitoneum indicates a ruptured ectopic pregnancy, which is a contraindication for methotrexate and requires surgical intervention.

SBA 69
b) Methotrexate therapy
Explanation: A stable patient with an adnexal mass and

positive β-hCG level is a candidate for methotrexate therapy.

SBA 70
e) Endometrial cavity
Explanation: Ectopic pregnancies occur outside the endometrial cavity, making it the least likely location for an ectopic pregnancy.

SBA 71

- **Answer**: b) Ectopic pregnancy
    - **Explanation**: An empty uterus with a positive pregnancy test and pelvic pain suggests an ectopic pregnancy.

SBA 72

- **Answer**: c) Laparoscopic salpingectomy
    - **Explanation**: Hemodynamically stable patients with an ectopic pregnancy and complex adnexal mass often require surgical management.

SBA 73

- **Answer**: d) History

SBA 74

- **Answer**: b) Methotrexate therapy
    - **Explanation**: Methotrexate is appropriate for stable patients with an unruptured ectopic pregnancy, a β-hCG level under

5000 IU/L, and an adnexal mass under 35 mm without fetal cardiac activity.

SBA 75

- **Answer**: a) Cervical ectopic pregnancy
  - **Explanation**: A gestational sac in the cervix indicates a cervical ectopic pregnancy, a rare but serious condition.

SBA 76

- **Answer**: b) Crown-rump length (CRL)
  - **Explanation**: CRL is the most accurate method for dating a pregnancy up to 13+6 weeks.

SBA 77

- **Answer**: d) Repeat ultrasound in 7 days
  - **Explanation**: If no heartbeat is detected and the CRL is below 7 mm, repeating the ultrasound in 7 days is recommended to confirm viability.

SBA 78

- **Answer**: e) Complex adnexal mass separate from the ovary
  - **Explanation**: A complex adnexal mass separate from the ovary strongly suggests an ectopic pregnancy.

SBA 79

- **Answer**: c) Repeat β-hCG in 48 hours
  - **Explanation**: Repeating the β-hCG in 48 hours helps assess whether the pregnancy is viable, especially when an ultrasound shows an empty uterus.

SBA 80

- **Answer**: c) Expectant management with follow-up if bleeding persists
    - **Explanation**: With a viable intrauterine pregnancy, expectant management is appropriate, with follow-up if symptoms worsen.

SBA 81

- **Answer**: d) Caesarean section scar ectopic pregnancy
    - **Explanation**: A gestational sac in the lower uterine segment, particularly near a previous cesarean scar, suggests a scar ectopic pregnancy.

SBA 82

- **Answer**: c) Laparoscopic cornual resection
    - **Explanation**: Cornual pregnancies often require surgical management due to the risk of rupture.

SBA 83

- **Answer**: c) Immediate laparoscopy
    - **Explanation**: Signs of rupture, such as severe abdominal pain, hypotension, and free fluid, necessitate immediate laparoscopy to address a possible ruptured ectopic pregnancy.

SBA 84

- **Answer**: b) Ampulla of the fallopian tube
    - **Explanation**: The ampulla is the most common site of implantation in an ectopic pregnancy.

SBA 85

- **Answer**: c) Early transvaginal ultrasound
  - **Explanation**: Early transvaginal ultrasound is the most accurate method for confirming intrauterine pregnancy, especially in women with a history of ectopic pregnancy.

SBA 86

- **Answer**: b) Methotrexate therapy
  - **Explanation**: Methotrexate is appropriate for stable patients with a β-hCG level under 5000 IU/L and an unruptured ectopic pregnancy.

SBA 87

- **Answer**: c) Heterotopic pregnancy
  - **Explanation**: A viable intrauterine pregnancy with free fluid in the abdomen suggests a possible concurrent ectopic pregnancy, known as a heterotopic pregnancy.

SBA 88

- **Answer**: c) Serial β-hCG measurements
  - **Explanation**: Serial β-hCG measurements help determine whether the pregnancy is progressing normally or if there is a risk of miscarriage or ectopic pregnancy.

SBA 89

- **Answer**: c) Expectant management
  - **Explanation**: Expectant management is recommended for a viable pregnancy with

a subchorionic hematoma, as most cases resolve on their own.

SBA 90

- **Answer**: e) Transvaginal ultrasound
    - **Explanation**: Transvaginal ultrasound is the best investigation to rule out an ectopic pregnancy, especially with a history of tubal surgery.

SBA 91

- **Answer**: c) Surgical evacuation
    - **Explanation**: Surgical evacuation is necessary when there are retained products of conception in the uterus after a miscarriage.

SBA 92

- **Answer**: b) Methotrexate therapy
    - **Explanation**: Methotrexate can be considered for a caesarean section scar ectopic pregnancy, depending on the size and β-hCG levels.

SBA 93

- **Answer**: c) Surgical evacuation
    - **Explanation**: Surgical evacuation is necessary when there is no heartbeat in a fetal pole measuring 25 mm, indicating a missed miscarriage.

SBA 94

- **Answer**: b) Threatened miscarriage
    - **Explanation**: A small subchorionic hemorrhage with a viable fetus is

associated with a threatened miscarriage, but many of these pregnancies continue to term.

SBA 95

- **Answer**: b) Reassess with ultrasound in 7 days
    - **Explanation**: When no heartbeat is visible with a CRL of 5 mm, reassessment in 7 days is appropriate to confirm viability.

SBA 96

- **Answer**: b) Missed miscarriage
    - **Explanation**: A CRL of 15 mm without a heartbeat indicates a missed miscarriage.

SBA 97

- **Answer**: c) Reassess with ultrasound in 7 days
    - **Explanation**: A large gestational sac with no fetal pole suggests a possible anembryonic pregnancy, and reassessment with ultrasound is recommended.

SBA 98

- **Answer**: b) Patient's preference
    - **Explanation**: The choice between medical and surgical management of a missed miscarriage often depends on the patient's preference after discussing options.

SBA 99

- **Answer**: c) Expectant management

- Explanation: Most subchorionic hemorrhages resolve without intervention, so expectant management is appropriate.

SBA 100

- **Answer**: b) Reassess with ultrasound in 7 days
  - **Explanation**: An empty gestational sac at 5 weeks with a mean diameter of 18 mm should be reassessed with ultrasound in 7 days to confirm viability.

SBA 101

- **Answer**: b) Heterotopic pregnancy
  - **Explanation**: A complex adnexal mass with an intrauterine gestational sac suggests a heterotopic pregnancy.

SBA 102

- **Answer**: c) Reassess with ultrasound in 7 days
  - **Explanation**: An ultrasound showing no heartbeat with a CRL of 8 mm warrants a follow-up scan in 7 days to confirm the findings.

SBA 103

- **Answer**: b) Missed miscarriage
  - **Explanation**: A gestational sac with a CRL of 7 mm and no heartbeat is indicative of a missed miscarriage.

SBA 104

- **Answer**: c) Surgical evacuation
  - **Explanation**: Surgical evacuation is indicated when there are retained products of conception in the uterus.

SBA 105

- **Answer**: a) Threatened miscarriage
  - **Explanation**: A viable intrauterine pregnancy with spotting and free fluid in the pouch of Douglas is likely a threatened miscarriage.

SBA 106

- **Answer**: c) Surgical evacuation
  - **Explanation**: A gestational sac with a fetal pole measuring 20 mm without a heartbeat indicates a missed miscarriage, typically managed surgically.

SBA 107

- **Answer**: b) Reassess with ultrasound in 7 days
  - **Explanation**: If no fetal pole is seen at 6 weeks, a follow-up ultrasound is recommended in 7 days.

SBA 108

- **Answer**: d) Surgical evacuation
  - **Explanation**: Heavy vaginal bleeding with retained gestational sac without a heartbeat requires surgical evacuation.

SBA 109

- **Answer**: c) Heterotopic pregnancy
  - **Explanation**: A viable intrauterine pregnancy with lower abdominal pain and free fluid may suggest a heterotopic pregnancy.

SBA 110

- **Answer**: b) Ectopic pregnancy
    - **Explanation**: An empty uterus with a complex adnexal mass is highly suggestive of an ectopic pregnancy.

SBA 111

- **Answer**: b) Reassess with ultrasound in 7 days
    - **Explanation**: If no heartbeat is detected in a CRL of 8 mm, a follow-up ultrasound in 7 days is recommended.

SBA 112

- **Answer**: b) Missed miscarriage
    - **Explanation**: A large gestational sac without a fetal pole indicates a missed miscarriage.

SBA 113

- **Answer**: c) Surgical evacuation
    - **Explanation**: Surgical evacuation is recommended when there are retained products of conception after a miscarriage.

SBA 114

- **Answer**: b) Ectopic pregnancy
    - **Explanation**: Severe pelvic pain with an empty uterus and adnexal mass at 7 weeks gestation suggests an ectopic pregnancy.

SBA 115:

- **Answer:** C) Ampullary section of the fallopian tube
  Explanation: The ampullary section of the fallopian tube is the most common site of ectopic pregnancy implantation, accounting for about 80% of cases.

SBA 116:

- **Answer: B) 11 in 1000**
  Explanation: The incidence of ectopic pregnancy in the UK is approximately 11 per 1000 pregnancies.

SBA 117:

Answer: C) Methotrexate administration
Explanation: Methotrexate is suitable for a stable patient with a small ectopic mass and β-hCG levels typically under 5000 IU/L, as in this case.

SBA 118:

Answer: C) 33%
Explanation: Approximately one-third (33%) of ectopic pregnancies occur without any known risk factors.

SBA 119:
Answer: B) Previous ectopic pregnancy
Explanation: A history of a previous ectopic pregnancy is the most significant risk factor for recurrence.

SBA 120:
Answer: A) Perform a serum β-hCG test
Explanation: In the context of an empty uterus on ultrasound, a serum β-hCG test is essential to assess for a possible ectopic pregnancy.

SBA 121:
Answer: a) Anti-D 250 IU
Explanation: Anti-D is recommended for Rh D-negative women experiencing a miscarriage at or above 12 weeks gestation.

SBA 122:
Answer: d) 500 IU
Explanation: Procedures like amniocentesis require a higher dose of anti-D prophylaxis (500 IU) in Rh D-negative women.

SBA 123:
Answer: c) No anti-D required
Explanation: Anti-D is not required for complete miscarriage below 12 weeks gestation without any risk factors.

SBA 124:
Answer: c) Anti-D 250 IU
Explanation: CVS is a procedure that necessitates 250 IU of anti-D prophylaxis.

SBA 125:
Answer: b) Administer 500 IU anti-D
Explanation: Trauma during pregnancy can cause fetal-maternal haemorrhage, requiring 500 IU anti-D.

SBA 126:
Answer: c) 500 IU
Explanation: Threatened miscarriage after 12 weeks requires 500 IU of anti-D.

SBA 127:
Answer: b) Administer 500 IU anti-D
Explanation: Antepartum haemorrhage after 12 weeks gestation requires 500 IU anti-D.

SBA 128:
Answer: c) 500 IU
Explanation: External cephalic version is a potentially sensitising event, requiring 500 IU of anti-D.

SBA 129:
Answer: a) Kleihauer-Betke test
Explanation: This test is used to quantify fetal-maternal haemorrhage.

SBA 130:
Answer: c) 1500 IU
Explanation: Routine Caesarean section after 20 weeks gestation requires 1500 IU of anti-D prophylaxis.

SBA 131:
Answer: c) 500 IU
Explanation: Surgical management of ectopic pregnancy requires 500 IU of anti-D prophylaxis.

SBA 132:
Answer: b) 500 IU
Explanation: A therapeutic abortion at or after 12 weeks gestation requires 500 IU of anti-D prophylaxis to prevent Rh sensitisation.

SBA 133:
Answer: d) Perform a Kleihauer-Betke test
Explanation: In cases of significant abdominal trauma, a Kleihauer-Betke test is indicated to quantify fetal-maternal haemorrhage, and the anti-D dose should be adjusted accordingly.

SBA 134:
Answer: b) Administer 500 IU anti-D

Explanation: Antepartum haemorrhage after 12 weeks gestation requires 500 IU of anti-D prophylaxis to prevent sensitisation.

SBA 135:
Answer: e) No anti-D required
Explanation: Anti-D prophylaxis is generally not required for a threatened miscarriage below 12 weeks gestation unless there is significant bleeding or surgical intervention.

SBA 136:
Answer: b) Administer 500 IU anti-D
Explanation: Intrauterine fetal demise after 12 weeks gestation necessitates the administration of 500 IU anti-D to prevent Rh sensitisation.

SBA 137:
Answer: b) 500 IU
Explanation: For any sensitising event, such as vaginal bleeding in the second trimester with an ongoing pregnancy, 500 IU of anti-D is required.

SBA 138:
Answer: c) 500 IU
Explanation: Amniocentesis after 20 weeks gestation requires 500 IU of anti-D to prevent Rh sensitisation.

SBA 139:
Answer: c) 1500 IU
Explanation: A routine Caesarean section at term for a Rh D-negative woman requires 1500 IU of anti-D prophylaxis.

SBA 140:
Answer: d) Perform a Kleihauer-Betke test
Explanation: Following significant abdominal trauma in the third trimester, a Kleihauer-Betke test is necessary to assess the amount of fetal-maternal haemorrhage, and the anti-D dose should be adjusted based on the results.

SBA 141:
Answer: c) Maternal age
Explanation: Maternal age is a significant risk factor for recurrent miscarriage, particularly in women aged 35 years and older.

SBA 142:
Answer: d) 50%
Explanation: The risk of miscarriage in women aged 40 years is approximately 50%, increasing significantly with age.

SBA 143:
Answer: b) Male partner's age
Explanation: Paternal age over 40 years is associated with an increased risk of miscarriage due to possible genetic abnormalities in sperm.

SBA 144:
Answer: b) Septate uterus
Explanation: A septate uterus is the most commonly associated uterine anomaly with recurrent miscarriage.

SBA 145:
Answer: c) 30-57%
Explanation: Chromosomal abnormalities are found in 30-57% of products of conception in recurrent miscarriage cases.

SBA 146:
Answer: c) Antiphospholipid syndrome
Explanation: Antiphospholipid syndrome is strongly associated with an increased risk of recurrent miscarriage and is treatable.

SBA 147:
Answer: b) Antiphospholipid antibody testing

Explanation: Antiphospholipid antibody testing is a key initial investigation in recurrent miscarriage.

SBA 148:
Answer: b) Hysteroscopic resection of the septum
Explanation: Hysteroscopic resection is recommended for women with recurrent miscarriage and a septate uterus.

SBA 149:
Answer: c) Serial cervical length monitoring with cerclage if needed
Explanation: Serial cervical length monitoring is the preferred management in suspected cervical insufficiency, with cerclage if needed.

SBA 150:
Answer: c) Thrombophilia screen
Explanation: A thrombophilia screen is appropriate in the next step of investigations for recurrent miscarriage after ruling out genetic causes.

SBA 151: Answer: b) Aspirin and low-molecular-weight heparin (LMWH)

Explanation: The combination of low-dose aspirin and LMWH is the first-line treatment for women with recurrent miscarriage associated with antiphospholipid syndrome, significantly improving live birth rates.

SBA 152: Answer: c) 75%

Explanation: Women with unexplained recurrent miscarriage have about a 75% chance of a successful pregnancy with supportive care alone.

SBA 153: Answer: a) Referral for preimplantation genetic diagnosis

Explanation: Preimplantation genetic diagnosis (PGD) is recommended for couples with a balanced translocation to reduce the risk of miscarriage associated with chromosomal abnormalities.

SBA 154: Answer: c) Trisomy 16

Explanation: Trisomy 16 is the most commonly identified chromosomal abnormality in the products of conception in cases of recurrent miscarriage.

SBA 155: Answer: b) Low-dose aspirin and low-molecular-weight heparin

Explanation: For women with antiphospholipid syndrome, the combination of low-dose aspirin and LMWH is the most appropriate treatment during pregnancy to reduce the risk of miscarriage.

SBA 156: Answer: b) As soon as pregnancy is confirmed

Explanation: LMWH therapy should be initiated as soon as pregnancy is confirmed in women with recurrent miscarriage and antiphospholipid syndrome to improve pregnancy outcomes.

SBA 157: Answer: e) 93%

Explanation: The risk of miscarriage in women aged 45 years or older is approximately 93%, highlighting the significant impact of advanced maternal age on pregnancy outcomes.

SBA 158: Answer: c) Reassurance and expectant management **Explanation:** In cases of unexplained recurrent miscarriage with normal investigations, reassurance and expectant management are appropriate, as many women can achieve a successful pregnancy.

SBA 159: Answer: c) Trisomy 16
Explanation: Trisomy 16 is the most common chromosomal condition found in the products of conception in women with recurrent miscarriage and normal parental karyotypes.

SBA 160: Answer: c) Low-dose aspirin and low-molecular-weight heparin
Explanation: The combination of low-dose aspirin and LMWH is the first-line treatment for recurrent miscarriage in women with diagnosed antiphospholipid syndrome.

SBA 161: e) 90%
NVP affects up to 90% of pregnant women, making it a common condition in pregnancy.

SBA 162: b) Hyperemesis gravidarum
The presentation of severe nausea, vomiting, weight loss, and dehydration is consistent with Hyperemesis Gravidarum.

SBA 163: b) GDF15 variants
Genetic variants associated with GDF15 are the greatest genetic risk factor for HG and its recurrence.

SBA 164: c) 9 weeks
NVP typically peaks around the 9th week of gestation.

SBA 165: d) Ondansetron
Ondansetron is considered a second-line treatment for NVP, not a first-line option.

SBA 166: e) All of the above
HG is associated with ketonuria, elevated thyroid function tests, elevated liver enzymes, and persistent vomiting causing weight loss and dehydration.

SBA 167: c) Ondansetron
Ondansetron is recommended as a second-line therapy for Hyperemesis Gravidarum.

SBA 168: b) Use corticosteroids
Corticosteroids are reserved for cases where standard therapies have been ineffective.

SBA 169: a) Normal saline with potassium chloride for hydration
Normal saline with potassium chloride is recommended for intravenous hydration in women with HG.

SBA 170: e) 3.6%
Hyperemesis Gravidarum affects between 0.3% and 3.6% of pregnancies.

SBA 171: d) Ketonuria
Ketonuria is not a reliable indicator of dehydration in pregnancy.

SBA 172: a) Thiamine supplementation
Thiamine supplementation should be provided, particularly before administering dextrose or parenteral nutrition in women with HG.

SBA 173: c) Small-for-gestational-age babies
HG is associated with risks of low birth weight and small-for-gestational-age babies.

SBA 174: b) It is linked with increased risks of postnatal depression
HG can severely impact a woman's quality of life and is linked with increased risks of postnatal depression.

SBA 175: b) It is recommended for short-term use only due to safety concerns
Ondansetron is recommended for short-term use due to safety concerns, particularly in early pregnancy.

SBA 176: b) Once the symptoms improve and she can maintain oral intake
Antiemetic treatment is typically stopped once the symptoms of HG improve, and the woman can maintain oral intake.

SBA 177: a) Pyridoxine-doxylamine
Pyridoxine-doxylamine is a first-line treatment for mild NVP managed in the community.

SBA 178: b) Persistent vomiting with significant weight loss and dehydration
Hospitalization is most likely required for women with HG who have persistent vomiting, significant weight loss, and dehydration.

SBA 179: c) Electrolyte imbalances
Electrolyte imbalances are a common complication of Hyperemesis Gravidarum due to persistent vomiting.

SBA 180: e) Blood cultures

Blood cultures are least likely to be informative in the context of Hyperemesis Gravidarum (HG). HG is primarily a condition related to severe nausea and vomiting in pregnancy, and blood cultures are typically used to detect infections, which are not a primary concern in HG. Therefore, while other tests like serum electrolytes, liver function tests, and thyroid function tests are important to assess complications of HG, blood cultures are not routinely indicated.

SBA 181: b) 4–7 weeks
Nausea and vomiting in pregnancy typically begin between 4th and 7th weeks of gestation.

SBA 182: c) Pyridoxine-doxylamine
Pyridoxine-doxylamine is the first-line pharmacological treatment for managing mild to moderate nausea and vomiting in pregnancy.

SBA 183: b) Dehydration
Ketonuria in Hyperemesis Gravidarum primarily indicates dehydration due to severe vomiting.

SBA 184: b) Hypokalaemia
Hypokalaemia is a common abnormal laboratory finding in Hyperemesis Gravidarum, resulting from excessive vomiting.

SBA 185: a) Ondansetron
Ondansetron is typically used as a second-line antiemetic when first-line treatments fail.

SBA 186: b) Normal saline with potassium chloride
Normal saline with potassium chloride is recommended for rehydration in Hyperemesis Gravidarum to address electrolyte imbalances.

SBA 187: c) Post-traumatic stress disorder (PTSD)
Hyperemesis Gravidarum can lead to long-term psychological effects, including PTSD.

SBA 188: c) Pregnancy-Unique Quantification of Emesis (PUQE) score
The PUQE score is a key diagnostic tool for assessing the severity of nausea and vomiting in pregnancy.

SBA 189: c) Previous history of Hyperemesis Gravidarum
A previous history of Hyperemesis Gravidarum is the

strongest predictor for its recurrence in future pregnancies.

SBA 190: b) Ginger supplements
Ginger supplements are often recommended as a non-pharmacological approach for managing mild nausea and vomiting in pregnancy.

SBA 191: d) 20 weeks
Hyperemesis Gravidarum most commonly resolves by 20 weeks of gestation in affected women.

SBA 192: d) Fetal macrosomia
Fetal macrosomia is not commonly associated with Hyperemesis Gravidarum; rather, low birth weight and nutritional deficiencies are more likely.

SBA 193: d) Referral to a specialist or hospital admission
Severe cases of Hyperemesis Gravidarum should be managed with specialist care, often requiring hospital admission.

SBA 194: b) Small, frequent meals
Small, frequent meals are commonly recommended to manage symptoms of nausea and vomiting in pregnancy.

SBA 195: c) Ketonuria
Although ketonuria is often present in Hyperemesis Gravidarum, it is not a definitive indicator of dehydration.

SBA 196: b) When oral intake is severely limited and other treatments have failed
Parenteral nutrition is considered when oral intake is inadequate, and other interventions have not been successful.

SBA 197: c) To prevent Wernicke's encephalopathy
Thiamine supplementation is critical in Hyperemesis

Gravidarum to prevent Wernicke's encephalopathy, especially before administering dextrose.

SBA 198: a) Postnatal depression
Severe Hyperemesis Gravidarum is associated with an increased risk of postnatal depression.

SBA 199: b) Significant weight loss
Significant weight loss would typically require further inpatient care, making it an unlikely discharge criterion.

SBA 200: b) 0.3%

Extended Match Questions (EMQ) Answers

EMQ 1: Diagnostic Approach in Pregnancy of Unknown Location (PUL)

1. B) Serial serum hCG measurements
2. B) Serial serum hCG measurements
3. D) Laparoscopy
4. A) Immediate transvaginal ultrasound
5. B) Serial serum hCG measurements

Explanation:
Serial hCG measurements are essential in cases of PUL to determine the trend and guide further management. Laparoscopy may be needed in cases with free fluid, indicating possible ectopic pregnancy.

EMQ 2: Management of Ectopic Pregnancy in the Context of PUL

1. E) Immediate surgical intervention
2. D) Repeat serum hCG in 48 hours
3. A) Methotrexate therapy
4. B) Laparoscopic salpingectomy
5. C) Expectant management

Explanation:
Management depends on clinical symptoms, hCG levels, and ultrasound findings. Immediate surgery is needed for

high-risk cases, while methotrexate or expectant management may be suitable for stable patients.

EMQ 3: Referral and Follow-up in Early Pregnancy Assessment Services

1. D) Routine antenatal care
2. A) Immediate referral to a senior gynaecologist
3. C) Urgent referral to early pregnancy assessment service
4. B) Follow-up scan in 7 days
5. D) Routine antenatal care

Explanation:
Routine antenatal care is appropriate for confirmed viable pregnancies. Urgent referral and follow-up are necessary for cases with concerning symptoms or unclear ultrasound findings.

EMQ 4: Criteria for Self-Referral to Early Pregnancy Assessment Services

1. B) Recurrent miscarriage
2. C) History of molar pregnancy
3. A) Previous ectopic pregnancy
4. D) No self-referral, requires professional assessment first
5. D) No self-referral, requires professional assessment first

Explanation:
Women with specific histories like recurrent miscarriage,

previous ectopic pregnancy, or molar pregnancy can self-refer to early pregnancy services.

EMQ 5: Investigations for Suspected Ectopic Pregnancy

1. A) Transvaginal ultrasound
2. B) Serum hCG measurement
3. D) Diagnostic laparoscopy
4. D) Diagnostic laparoscopy
5. A) Transvaginal ultrasound

Explanation:
Transvaginal ultrasound and serum hCG measurements are crucial first-line investigations. Laparoscopy is indicated when clinically indicated either with ultrasound scan and/or clinical assessment confirming a disturbed ectopic pregnancy.

EMQ 6: Referral Criteria to Early Pregnancy Assessment Services (EPAS)

1. A) History of ectopic pregnancy
2. C) Recurrent miscarriage
3. E) History of molar pregnancy
4. D) Professional assessment required before referral
5. D) Professional assessment required before referral

EMQ 7: Initial Management of Pregnancy of Unknown Location (PUL)

1. A) Serial serum hCG measurement
2. A) Serial serum hCG measurement
3. E) Diagnostic laparoscopy
4. E) Diagnostic laparoscopy
5. A) Serial serum hCG measurement

EMQ 8: Risk Factors for Ectopic Pregnancy

1. C) Pelvic inflammatory disease (PID)
2. B) Tubal surgery
3. A) Previous ectopic pregnancy
4. D) Use of intrauterine contraceptive device (IUCD)
5. E) Previous molar pregnancy

EMQ 9: Follow-up in Early Pregnancy Assessment Services

1. D) Routine antenatal care
2. A) Immediate referral to senior gynaecologist
3. B) Repeat serum hCG in 48 hours
4. C) Follow-up scan in 7 days
5. A) Immediate referral to senior gynaecologist

EMQ 10: Interpretation of Serum hCG Levels in PUL

1. D) Repeat hCG in 48 hours
2. B) Ectopic pregnancy likely
3. C) Pregnancy failing (PUL)
4. B) Ectopic pregnancy likely
5. D) Repeat hCG in 48 hours

EMQ 11

Answers:

a) Tubal surgery - Tubal ligation is a significant risk factor for ectopic pregnancy due to the potential for tubal damage.

c) Smoking - Smoking is a known risk factor, likely due to its effects on ciliary function within the fallopian tubes.

d) In vitro fertilization (IVF) - IVF increases the risk of ectopic pregnancy, especially due to the manipulation of embryos.

b) Pelvic inflammatory disease (PID) - PID can cause scarring and damage to the fallopian tubes, increasing ectopic pregnancy risk.

e) No known risk factors - A significant proportion of women with ectopic pregnancies have no identifiable risk factors.

EMQ 12

Answers:

1. **a) Ampullary section of the fallopian tube** - This is the most common site of ectopic pregnancy.
2. **e) Cervix** - Cervical ectopic pregnancies are rare but can occur and are associated with significant morbidity.
3. **c) Fimbriae end of the fallopian tube** - Ectopic pregnancies can occur here, though less commonly.
4. **b) Isthmus** - Ectopic pregnancies in the isthmus can cause significant complications.
5. **d) Interstitial part of the fallopian tube** - Interstitial pregnancies are rarer but more dangerous due to the risk of uterine rupture.

EMQ 13

Answers:

1. **a) Abdominal or pelvic pain** - This is the most common presenting symptom of ectopic pregnancy.
2. **b) Vaginal bleeding** - Often seen in conjunction with other symptoms like pain.
3. **e) Syncope** - Dizziness and fainting can indicate haemorrhage in a ruptured ectopic pregnancy.
4. **d) Shoulder tip pain** - Indicative of referred pain due to diaphragmatic irritation from intra-abdominal bleeding.
5. **c) Amenorrhoea** - A classic symptom of early pregnancy, including ectopic pregnancy.

EMQ 14

Answers:

1. **b) Complex adnexal mass** - Indicative of an ectopic pregnancy, especially if seen on transvaginal ultrasound.

2. **e) Pseudogestational sac in the uterus** - A sign of ectopic pregnancy, often seen in conjunction with other findings.
3. **d) Gestational sac with yolk sac in adnexa** - A definitive sign of ectopic pregnancy.
4. **c) Free fluid in the pelvis** - Suggestive of ruptured ectopic pregnancy with hemoperitoneum.
5. **a) Empty uterus** - In the presence of a positive pregnancy test, an empty uterus can suggest an ectopic pregnancy.

EMQ 15

Answers:

1. **a) Methotrexate** - Suitable for a stable patient with low β-hCG and small, unruptured ectopic pregnancy.
2. **e) Laparotomy** - Required in cases of haemodynamic instability and ruptured ectopic pregnancy.
3. **b) Expectant management** - Appropriate in cases of resolving ectopic pregnancies with falling β-hCG.
4. **c) Salpingectomy** - The removal of the affected tube is indicated when the contralateral tube is healthy.
5. **d) Salpingotomy** - Indicated in women with only one tube or with fertility concerns.

EMQ 16

Answers:

1. **b) Ampullary** - The ampullary region is the most common site of ectopic pregnancies.
2. **a) Cervical** - Cervical ectopic pregnancies are rare and can present with heavy bleeding.

3. **c) Isthmic** - Ectopic pregnancies in the isthmus can be particularly dangerous due to the narrow lumen.
4. **d) Fimbrial** - Fimbrial ectopic pregnancies occur at the distal end of the fallopian tube.
5. **e) Interstitial** - Interstitial pregnancies occur at the junction of the fallopian tube and uterus and carry a high risk of rupture.

EMQ 17

Answers:

1. **a) Prior ectopic pregnancy** - A previous ectopic pregnancy is a significant risk factor for recurrence.
2. **d) Pelvic inflammatory disease (PID)** - PID increases the risk due to tubal scarring.
3. **b) Intrauterine device (IUD) use** - While IUDs reduce the overall risk of pregnancy, if pregnancy occurs, the risk of it being ectopic is higher.
4. **c) Tubal surgery** - Surgery on the fallopian tubes increases the risk of ectopic pregnancy due to potential damage.
5. **e) No identifiable risk factor** - Many ectopic pregnancies occur without any known risk factors.

EMQ 18

Answers:

1. **a) Repeat β-hCG in 48 hours** - Essential to confirm the effectiveness of methotrexate treatment.
2. **c) Urine pregnancy test in 3 weeks** - Follow-up after salpingectomy to ensure the resolution of pregnancy tissue.

3. **b) Weekly β-hCG until <20 IU/L** - Required after salpingotomy to ensure all ectopic tissue is resolved.
4. **d) Immediate laparoscopy** - Required in cases of persistent pain or concern for rupture.
5. **e) MRI assessment** - Used in complex cases such as interstitial ectopic pregnancy for better visualization.

EMQ 19

Answers:

1. **a) Hemodynamically stable with low β-hCG (<1500 IU/L)** - Ideal candidate for methotrexate therapy.
2. **b) Unruptured ectopic pregnancy with a mass smaller than 35 mm** - A criterion for methotrexate treatment.
3. **d) Presence of fetal cardiac activity** - Typically contraindicates the use of methotrexate due to lower efficacy.
4. **e) Tubal rupture with haemodynamic instability** - Requires immediate surgical intervention, not methotrexate.
5. **b) Unruptured ectopic pregnancy with a mass smaller than 35 mm** - Suitable for methotrexate.

EMQ 20

Answers:

1. **a) Systemic methotrexate** - Suitable for a cervical ectopic pregnancy with low β-hCG and no cardiac activity.
2. **c) Surgical management due to life-threatening bleeding** - Necessary when significant haemorrhage is present.

3. **e) Methotrexate with intra-amniotic injection** - May improve outcomes in cases with higher β-hCG or fetal cardiac activity.

EMQ 21:

1. D) Repeat ultrasound in 7 days
2. C) Medical management with misoprostol
3. A) Expectant management
4. E) Reassurance and routine antenatal care
5. F) Laparoscopy

Explanation:

- A repeat ultrasound in 7 days is indicated if the CRL is less than 7 mm with no heartbeat.
- Medical management is preferred for managing incomplete miscarriages.
- Expectant management can be considered if there is no immediate risk, such as heavy bleeding or infection.
- Reassurance and routine antenatal care are appropriate when a heartbeat is detected.
- Laparoscopy is necessary for suspected ectopic pregnancies.

EMQ 22:

1. E) Repeat ultrasound in 7 days
2. A) Expectant management
3. E) Repeat ultrasound in 7 days
4. G) Immediate referral to early pregnancy assessment service
5. C) Reassurance and routine antenatal care

Explanation:

- Repeat ultrasound is required when a CRL is <7 mm without a visible heartbeat.
- Expectant management is appropriate for a confirmed intrauterine pregnancy with mild symptoms.
- Immediate referral is needed for potentially serious complications, such as suspected ectopic pregnancy.

EMQ 23:

1. A) Repeat ultrasound in 7 days
2. A) Repeat ultrasound in 7 days
3. F) Laparoscopy
4. A) Repeat ultrasound in 7 days
5. C) Reassurance and routine antenatal care

Explanation:

- Repeat scans are essential when there is uncertainty in early pregnancy assessments.
- Laparoscopy is indicated for ectopic pregnancy suspicion.
- Routine care is recommended when a heartbeat is present.

EMQ 24:

1. G) Reassurance and routine antenatal care
2. B) Repeat ultrasound in 7 days
3. A) Serial β-hCG measurement
4. D) Laparoscopy
5. B) Repeat ultrasound in 7 days

Explanation:

- Routine care with reassurance is necessary when there is no significant risk.
- A repeat ultrasound is useful for further assessment of uncertain findings.
- Serial β-hCG helps monitor progress when the initial scan is inconclusive.

EMQ 25:

1. D) Repeat ultrasound in 7 days
2. C) Surgical management
3. F) Laparoscopy
4. B) Surgical management
5. E) Reassurance and routine antenatal care

Explanation:

- A follow-up scan is advised when findings are unclear.
- Surgical management is necessary for cases of confirmed miscarriage with retained products.
- Laparoscopy is indicated for severe symptoms with suspected ectopic pregnancy.

EMQ 26:

1. B) Repeat ultrasound in 7 days
2. C) Expectant management
3. B) Repeat ultrasound in 7 days
4. D) Laparoscopy
5. G) Reassurance and routine antenatal care

Explanation:

- Repeat ultrasound is appropriate if there is uncertainty, such as an absent heartbeat in a small CRL.
- Expectant management is suitable when there are mild symptoms and no immediate intervention is needed.
- Laparoscopy is indicated for suspected ectopic pregnancy.
- Reassurance and routine care are recommended when a heartbeat is confirmed.

EMQ 27:

1. A) Repeat ultrasound in 7 days
2. D) Surgical management
3. B) Laparoscopy
4. E) Reassurance and routine antenatal care
5. D) Surgical management

Explanation:

- Repeat ultrasound is useful when there's a possibility of delayed diagnosis.
- Surgical management is necessary for cases of missed or incomplete miscarriage.
- Laparoscopy is indicated for complex adnexal masses or severe pain with suspected ectopic pregnancy.

EMQ 28:

1. F) Repeat ultrasound in 7 days
2. A) Surgical management
3. B) Laparoscopy
4. E) Reassurance and routine antenatal care
5. F) Repeat ultrasound in 7 days

Explanation:

- A follow-up scan is essential when the CRL is small without a visible heartbeat.
- Surgical management is required for heavy bleeding with a significant risk of miscarriage.
- Laparoscopy is necessary for diagnosing and managing suspected ectopic pregnancies.

EMQ 29:

1. D) Surgical management
2. F) Reassurance and routine antenatal care
3. E) Laparoscopy
4. A) Serial β-hCG measurement
5. D) Surgical management

Explanation:

- Surgical management is appropriate when there's a significant likelihood of non-viability.
- Routine care is recommended when there's no immediate risk and a heartbeat is detected.
- Serial β-hCG helps monitor cases where ultrasound findings are inconclusive.

EMQ 30:

1. D) Repeat ultrasound in 7 days
2. B) Surgical management
3. A) Laparoscopy
4. D) Repeat ultrasound in 7 days
5. E) Reassurance and routine antenatal care

Explanation:

- A repeat scan is needed when the initial findings are inconclusive.
- Surgical management is necessary for cases where there's an increased risk of complications.
- Laparoscopy is essential for diagnosing and managing complex adnexal masses.

EMQ 31:

1. A) Repeat ultrasound in 7 days
2. B) Surgical management
3. D) Laparoscopy
4. F) Reassurance and routine antenatal care
5. E) Serial β-hCG measurement

Explanation:

- Repeat ultrasound is indicated for a small CRL with no visible heartbeat.
- Surgical management is needed for large empty sacs with no fetal pole.
- Laparoscopy is essential for complex adnexal masses or suspected ectopic pregnancy.
- Reassurance is appropriate for confirmed viable pregnancies.

EMQ 32:

1. A) Repeat scan in 7 days
2. D) Surgical management
3. A) Repeat scan in 7 days

4. F) Expectant management
5. C) Serial β-hCG measurement

Explanation:

- A follow-up scan is needed when initial findings are inconclusive.
- Surgical management is necessary when there's a significant risk of complications.
- Serial β-hCG helps in monitoring when ultrasound findings are unclear.

EMQ 33:

1. F) Repeat ultrasound in 7 days
2. A) Surgical management
3. B) Laparoscopy
4. E) Reassurance and routine antenatal care
5. F) Repeat ultrasound in 7 days

Explanation:

- A repeat scan is essential for inconclusive CRL findings.
- Surgical management is required for heavy bleeding with a high risk of miscarriage.
- Laparoscopy is crucial for diagnosing and managing suspected ectopic pregnancies.

EMQ 34:

1. D) Repeat ultrasound in 7 days

2. B) Surgical management
3. F) Repeat ultrasound in 7 days
4. A) Laparoscopy
5. E) Reassurance and routine antenatal care

Explanation:

- A repeat scan is appropriate for inconclusive findings in early pregnancy.
- Surgical management is necessary for high-risk pregnancies.
- Laparoscopy is indicated for complex adnexal masses, especially with pain.

EMQ 35:

1. D) Surgical management
2. F) Medical management with misoprostol
3. A) Laparoscopy
4. C) Repeat ultrasound in 7 days
5. E) Reassurance and routine antenatal care

Explanation:

- Surgical management is necessary for high-risk cases with large empty sacs.
- Medical management is appropriate for early non-viable pregnancies.
- Laparoscopy is essential for suspected ectopic pregnancies with pain or adnexal mass.

EMQ 36:

1. E) Repeat ultrasound in 7 days
2. B) Surgical management
3. D) Laparoscopy
4. A) Serial β-hCG measurement
5. C) Expectant management

Explanation:

- A repeat ultrasound is indicated for inconclusive early pregnancy findings.
- Surgical management is necessary for high-risk pregnancies with large empty sacs.
- Laparoscopy is crucial for diagnosing and managing suspected ectopic pregnancies.
- Serial β-hCG measurement helps in monitoring early pregnancy with inconclusive ultrasound results.

EMQ 37:

1. D) Repeat ultrasound in 7 days
2. D) Repeat ultrasound in 7 days
3. F) Expectant management
4. A) Serial β-hCG measurement
5. C) Serial β-hCG measurement

Explanation:

- A repeat ultrasound is required for inconclusive CRL findings.

- Expectant management may be appropriate for non-viable pregnancies.
- Serial β-hCG measurement helps in monitoring early pregnancy when ultrasound findings are inconclusive.

EMQ 38:

1. F) Repeat ultrasound in 7 days
2. A) Surgical management
3. B) Laparoscopy
4. E) Reassurance and routine antenatal care
5. C) Medical management with misoprostol

Explanation:

- A repeat scan is necessary for non-confirmed early pregnancies.
- Surgical management is needed for large empty sacs with a high risk of complications.
- Laparoscopy is indicated for suspected ectopic pregnancies with complex adnexal masses.

EMQ 39:

1. F) Repeat ultrasound in 7 days
2. C) Surgical management
3. A) Laparoscopy
4. B) Serial β-hCG measurement
5. E) Reassurance and routine antenatal care

Explanation:

- A repeat ultrasound is appropriate for inconclusive CRL findings.
- Surgical management is required for high-risk pregnancies.
- Laparoscopy is essential for diagnosing and managing suspected ectopic pregnancies.

EMQ 40:

1. B) Surgical management
2. E) Repeat ultrasound in 7 days
3. C) Serial β-hCG measurement
4. A) Laparoscopy
5. F) Reassurance and routine antenatal care

Explanation:

- Surgical management is necessary for high-risk pregnancies with large sacs and no fetal pole.
- A repeat ultrasound is required for non-confirmed early pregnancies.
- Serial β-hCG measurement helps in monitoring early pregnancy when ultrasound findings are unclear.

EMQ41:

1. **b) Within 10 days** - Anti-D should be administered within 10 days if the 72-hour window is missed.

2. **a) Within 72 hours** - Administering Anti-D within 72 hours is appropriate.
3. **c) No anti-D required** - Anti-D is not generally required for missed miscarriage before 12 weeks with no bleeding.
4. **a) Within 72 hours** - Anti-D should be given within 72 hours after the procedure.
5. **c) No anti-D required** - Anti-D is not required for early spotting under 12 weeks without heavy bleeding.

EMQ42:

1. **c) 1500 IU** - Routine cesarean sections at term require 1500 IU of Anti-D.
2. **a) 250 IU** - The recommended dosage for a miscarriage under 12 weeks with bleeding is 250 IU.
3. **b) 500 IU** - Significant fetal-maternal haemorrhage after 20 weeks requires at least 500 IU, adjusted based on test results.
4. **d) No anti-D required** - Anti-D is not generally required for early spontaneous miscarriage without bleeding.
5. **b) 500 IU** - Therapeutic abortion after 12 weeks requires 500 IU of Anti-D.

EMQ43:

1. **a) Ectopic pregnancy managed surgically** - Anti-D is indicated after surgical management of an ectopic pregnancy.
2. **b) Threatened miscarriage under 12 weeks with no heavy bleeding** - Anti-D is not required for threatened miscarriage under 12 weeks with no heavy bleeding.
3. **e) Missed miscarriage at 15 weeks** - Anti-D is required for missed miscarriages over 12 weeks.
4. **d) Normal vaginal delivery at term** - Anti-D is needed after normal delivery at term.

5. **c) Amniocentesis** - Anti-D is indicated after amniocentesis.

EMQ44:

1. **a) Administer within 10 days** - Anti-D can still be effective if given within 10 days.
2. **a) Administer within 10 days** - Administering within 10 days is the appropriate course of action.
3. **e) Give higher dose of 1500 IU** - Administer a higher dose if the initial dose was insufficient.
4. **e) Give higher dose of 1500 IU** - Administer a higher dose since the 10-day window was exceeded.
5. **d) No further action required** - If Anti-D is given within 72 hours, no further action is needed.

EMQ45:

1. **c) External cephalic version** - Anti-D is required after external cephalic version.
2. **b) Antepartum haemorrhage after 20 weeks gestation** - Anti-D is needed after antepartum haemorrhage.
3. **c) External cephalic version** - Anti-D is required in this case.
4. **a) First trimester miscarriage with no bleeding** - Anti-D is not required.
5. **e) Therapeutic abortion at 8 weeks** - Anti-D is indicated after a therapeutic abortion, even at 8 weeks.

EMQ46:

1. **a) Therapeutic abortion at 9 weeks** - Anti-D is required after a therapeutic abortion, even if it is early in the pregnancy.
2. **b) Spontaneous miscarriage at 6 weeks without bleeding** - Anti-D is not required in this case.

3. **e) External cephalic version at 38 weeks** - Anti-D should be given after an external cephalic version.
4. **c) Amniocentesis at 16 weeks** - Anti-D is indicated after an amniocentesis.
5. **e) External cephalic version at 38 weeks** - Anti-D should be administered following the procedure.

EMQ47:

1. **b) 500 IU** - The recommended dose of Anti-D following amniocentesis at 18 weeks is 500 IU.
2. **b) 500 IU** - For a miscarriage with significant bleeding at 10 weeks, 500 IU of Anti-D is appropriate.
3. **b) 500 IU** - The appropriate dose for an external cephalic version at 32 weeks is 500 IU.
4. **a) 250 IU** - For an elective abortion at 9 weeks, the appropriate dose is 250 IU.
5. **d) 1500 IU** - For a cesarean section at term, the appropriate dose of Anti-D is 1500 IU.

EMQ48:

1. **a) Administer within 10 days** - Anti-D is still effective if administered within 10 days of the event.
2. **a) Administer within 10 days** - Anti-D should be administered within 10 days if the initial window is missed.
3. **e) Administer higher dose** - Administer a higher dose if the initial dose was insufficient.
4. **e) Administer higher dose** - The higher dose is necessary due to the delay beyond 10 days.
5. **a) Administer within 10 days** - Anti-D administered within 72 hours is still within the recommended timeframe.

EMQ49:

1. **b) Antepartum haemorrhage at 22 weeks** - Anti-D is required after antepartum haemorrhage.
2. **c) Ectopic pregnancy treated surgically** - Anti-D prophylaxis is needed after surgical management of an ectopic pregnancy.
3. **d) Spontaneous rupture of membranes at term** - Anti-D should be administered in this situation.
4. **e) Therapeutic abortion at 8 weeks** - Anti-D is indicated following a therapeutic abortion.
5. **a) First trimester miscarriage with bleeding** - Anti-D should be administered if there is bleeding.

EMQ50:

1. **c) Administer Anti-D within 10 days** - Administer within 10 days if the initial window is missed.
2. **c) Administer Anti-D within 10 days** - The appropriate management is to administer Anti-D within 10 days.
3. **c) Administer Anti-D within 10 days** - Administer within 10 days if the initial 72-hour window is missed.
4. **c) Administer Anti-D within 10 days** - Anti-D should be administered within 10 days if the initial timeframe is exceeded.
5. **a) No further action needed** - If Anti-D is given within 72 hours, no further action is required.

EMQ 51:

1. c) Testing for antiphospholipid antibodies
2. e) Hysteroscopy
3. c) Testing for antiphospholipid antibodies
4. a) Parental karyotyping

5. d) Testing for inherited thrombophilias

Explanation: These investigations are essential for diagnosing causes of recurrent miscarriage, guiding further management.

EMQ 52:

1. b) Hysteroscopic resection
2. e) Cervical cerclage
3. f) Combined hysteroscopy and laparoscopy
4. a) Expectant management
5. b) Hysteroscopic resection

Explanation: Appropriate management is crucial depending on the uterine anomaly and its impact on pregnancy outcomes.

EMQ 53:

1. a) Maternal age >35 years
2. c) Chromosomal anomalies
3. b) Smoking
4. e) Uterine structural anomalies
5. f) Obesity

Explanation: Various risk factors contribute to recurrent miscarriage, and identifying them is essential for targeted intervention.

EMQ 54:

1. a) Presence of antiphospholipid antibodies
2. b) History of a previous live birth
3. d) Recurrent miscarriage without identified cause

4. f) Presence of uterine anomaly
5. e) Increasing maternal age

Explanation: Prognostic factors determine the likelihood of a successful pregnancy and guide clinical management.

EMQ 55:

1. c) Antiphospholipid syndrome
2. a) Factor V Leiden mutation
3. d) Protein S deficiency
4. b) Prothrombin gene mutation
5. f) Antithrombin III deficiency

Explanation: Different types of thrombophilia are associated with recurrent miscarriage, and identifying them helps in providing appropriate prophylactic treatment.

EMQ 56:

1. a) Cervical incompetence
2. b) Uterine fibroids
3. c) Antiphospholipid syndrome
4. e) Septate uterus
5. d) Chromosomal abnormalities

Explanation: The causes of second-trimester miscarriage vary and can include structural, genetic, and immune factors.

EMQ 57:

1. a) Cervical cerclage

2. b) Progesterone supplementation
3. c) Expectant management
4. e) Hysteroscopic resection
5. f) Laparoscopic resection

Explanation: Management depends on the specific cause of cervical incompetence and associated factors.

EMQ 58:

1. a) Parental karyotyping
2. d) Cytogenetic analysis of products of conception
3. b) Genetic counselling
4. c) Preimplantation genetic diagnosis (PGD)
5. f) Testing for Factor V Leiden mutation

Explanation: Genetic investigations are crucial in diagnosing and planning treatment for recurrent miscarriage.

EMQ 59:

1. a) Early pregnancy assessment unit (EPAU)
2. c) Aspirin and heparin therapy
3. d) Cervical cerclage
4. b) Psychological support
5. f) Expectant management

Explanation: Supportive care is vital in managing recurrent miscarriage and can include medical, surgical, and psychological support.

EMQ 60:

1. d) Hyperprolactinemia

2. f) Luteal phase defect
3. c) Thyroid dysfunction
4. b) Polycystic Ovary Syndrome (PCOS)
5. e) Ovarian insufficiency

Explanation: Hormonal imbalances can play a significant role in recurrent miscarriage, and identifying these factors is essential for treatment.

EMQ 61

1. **a) Mild NVP** - Mild symptoms with no vomiting suggest mild NVP.
2. **c) Hyperemesis Gravidarum** - Severe vomiting and weight loss indicate HG.
3. **c) Hyperemesis Gravidarum** - Severe symptoms and dehydration are indicative of HG.
4. **b) Moderate NVP** - Mild to moderate symptoms suggest moderate NVP.
5. **d) Gastroenteritis** - Sudden onset of vomiting and diarrhoea with fever is more suggestive of gastroenteritis.

EMQ 62

1. **a) Reassurance and dietary advice** - Mild symptoms can be managed with reassurance and dietary advice.
2. **c) Hospital admission with intravenous fluids** - Severe dehydration requires hospitalisation and IV fluids.

3. **d) Nutritional support with enteral feeding** - Persistent symptoms and weight loss require nutritional support.

4. **e) Referral for psychiatric support** - Depression and anxiety in HG warrant psychiatric support.

5. **b) Antiemetic therapy** - Moderate symptoms not responding to dietary measures may require antiemetics.

EMQ 63

1. **c) History of HG in previous pregnancy** - A history of HG is a strong risk factor.

2. **b) Twin pregnancy** - Twin pregnancies increase the risk of HG.

3. **a) Nulliparity** - First-time pregnancies are a risk factor for NVP and HG.

4. **d) Obesity** - Obesity is associated with an increased risk of HG.

5. **e) Low socioeconomic status** - Lower socioeconomic status can be a risk factor for severe HG.

EMQ 64

1. **a) Electrolyte imbalance** - HG can cause hyponatremia and hypokalemia.

2. **b) Fetal growth restriction** - HG is associated with fetal growth restriction.

3. **c) Preterm delivery** - HG increases the risk of preterm delivery.

4. **d) Postnatal depression** - HG can lead to postnatal depression.

5. **e) Gestational diabetes** - Gestational diabetes, while not typically associated with HG, could occur independently.

EMQ 65

1. **c) Liver function tests** - Jaundice and elevated liver enzymes in HG patients require LFTs.

2. **a) Serum electrolytes** - Hypokalemia is common in severe HG.

3. **b) Thyroid function tests** - Suspected thyroid abnormalities require TFTs.

4. **d) Ultrasound scan** - An ultrasound scan is necessary to rule out molar pregnancy in HG.

5. **e) Urinalysis for ketones** - Ketones in urine indicate dehydration in HG.

EMQ 66

1. **d) Molar pregnancy** - Severe vomiting, weight loss, and larger-than-expected fundal height suggest a molar pregnancy.

2. **c) Pyelonephritis** - Nausea, vomiting, fever, and bacteriuria are indicative of pyelonephritis.

3. **e) Gallstones** - Elevated liver enzymes and right upper quadrant pain suggest gallstones.

4. **d) Molar pregnancy** - Absence of a fetal heartbeat and the presence of an abnormal mass on ultrasound suggest a molar pregnancy.

5. **b) Gastroenteritis** - Sudden onset of symptoms following food consumption suggests gastroenteritis.

EMQ 67

1. **c) Hospital admission** - Severe dehydration and persistent vomiting despite oral antiemetics necessitate hospital admission.

2. **b) Intravenous fluid replacement** - Severe vomiting and inability to maintain hydration require IV fluids.

3. **d) Thiamine supplementation** - Prolonged vomiting and poor nutrition put the patient at risk of Wernicke's encephalopathy, requiring thiamine.

4. **a) Oral rehydration therapy** - Mild symptoms can be managed with dietary modifications and oral hydration.

5. **e) Termination of pregnancy** - In severe, refractory cases of HG, where multiple therapies have failed, termination may be considered.

EMQ 68

1. **e) Family history of HG** - A strong family history is a significant risk factor for HG.

2. **b) Twin pregnancy** - Twin pregnancies increase the likelihood of HG.

3. **a) History of motion sickness** - A history of motion sickness is associated with an increased risk of NVP and HG.

4. **c) Advanced maternal age** - Older maternal age is associated with an increased risk of NVP.

5. **d) Female fetus** - Carrying a female fetus has been linked with a higher risk of HG.

EMQ 69

1. **b) Wernicke's encephalopathy** - Confusion, ataxia, and ophthalmoplegia in the context of HG suggest Wernicke's encephalopathy.

2. **c) Small for gestational age (SGA) infant** - HG is associated with an increased risk of delivering an SGA infant.

3. **a) Electrolyte imbalance** - Low potassium and sodium levels indicate an electrolyte imbalance, a common complication of HG.

4. **d) Post-traumatic stress disorder (PTSD)** - Anxiety and flashbacks related to pregnancy experience may suggest PTSD.

5. **e) Spontaneous abortion** - Persistent HG increases the risk of spontaneous miscarriage.

EMQ 70

1. **a) Pre-emptive use of antiemetics** - Pre-emptive antiemetics may reduce the risk of recurrence in subsequent pregnancies.

2. **e) Monitoring for postnatal depression** - Long-term mental health impact requires monitoring for postnatal depression.

3. **d) Nutritional counselling** - Adequate nutrition is essential, requiring dietary advice during HG.

4. **c) Psychological support** - Multiple hospital admissions and severe HG warrant psychological support.

5. **c) Psychological support** - A history of HG and postnatal depression necessitates close monitoring and support.

www.ingramcontent.com/pod-product-compliance
Lightning Source LLC
Chambersburg PA
CBHW052146220526
45471CB00004B/1542